UNDERSTANDING SPIRITUAL
and
PHYSICAL HEALTH

A BIBLICAL PERSPECTIVE

Troy A. Roberson

WESTBOW
PRESS®
A DIVISION OF THOMAS NELSON
& ZONDERVAN

Unless otherwise noted, Scripture quotations are taken from the King James Version, public domain.

Scripture quotations marked (AMP) are taken from the *Amplified Bible*, Copyright 2015 by The Lockman Foundation, La Habra, CA 90631. Used by permission. All rights reserved.

Scripture quotations marked (ESV) are taken from *The Holy Bible, English Standard Version*, Permanent Text Edition (2016). Copyright 2001 by Crossway Bibles, a publishing ministry of Good News Publishers. Used by permission. All rights reserved.

Scripture quotations marked (NIV) are taken from the *Holy Bible, New International Version*, NIV, Copyright 1973, 1978, 1984, 2011 by biblical, Inc. Used by permission. All rights reserved worldwide.

Scripture quotations marked (NKJV) are taken from the *New King James Version*. Copyright 1982 by Thomas Nelson, Inc. Used by permission. All rights reserved.

This book is a work of non-fiction. Unless otherwise noted, the author and the publisher make no explicit guarantees as to the accuracy of the information contained in this book and in some cases, names of people and places have been altered to protect their privacy.

WestBow Press books may be ordered through booksellers or by contacting:

WestBow Press
A Division of Thomas Nelson & Zondervan
1663 Liberty Drive
Bloomington, IN 47403
www.westbowpress.com
1 (866) 928-1240

Because of the dynamic nature of the Internet, any web addresses or links contained in this book may have changed since publication and may no longer be valid. The views expressed in this work are solely those of the author and do not necessarily reflect the views of the publisher, and the publisher hereby disclaims any responsibility for them.

Any people depicted in stock imagery provided by Thinkstock are models, and such images are being used for illustrative purposes only. Certain stock imagery © Thinkstock.

ISBN: 978-1-5127-9746-6 (sc)
ISBN: 978-1-5127-9745-9 (hc)
ISBN: 978-1-5127-9744-2 (e)

Library of Congress Control Number: 2017911714

Print information available on the last page.

WestBow Press rev. date: 12/15/2017

Contents

Acknowledgments

First, I want to thank the Lord Jesus Christ for inspiring me to write this book. On September 26, 2013, at 2:33 am, the Lord revealed to me the subject of health and wellness in our spiritual lives. Being led by the Spirit of God, it was my endeavor to respond writing a book about the need to develop our spirit, soul, and body in the spiritual principles in the Word of God. This book is to the glory of God for his loving mercies and blessing in my life through my Lord and Savior Jesus Christ.

I want to thank the greatest thing that ever happened to me is my beautiful wife Tonya, who has supported me from the beginning when I told her that the Lord inspired me to write about our spiritual and natural health that is essential to living a good life. I want to also thank God for our beautiful daughters, Victoria and Alivia, for bringing so much joy into our lives.

I want to thank my best friends, Audras and Patricia Nixon, who prayerfully supported me that the project would be successful. I will always be grateful for their words of encouragement.

I want to acknowledge some special people who had a major impact on teaching me the Word of God. First, I want to thank my mother, she raised me to know the Lord. She taught me to study the Word of God and was the first teacher of my spiritual development as a young man. I cannot forget my longtime friend, spiritual mentor, Ronald Childress, who taught me how to understand the scriptures and how to properly apply the text to my life. I want to thank my brothers and sisters who have always supported me: Marc, Curtis, Jimmy, Andre, Jason, Nicole and Natalie I love you all so much!!! I want to thank my longtime friends Donovan and Penny Gibbs. Two special friends who went home to be with the Lord, my spiritual mother Henrine Adams (Patricia Nixon's mother) she taught me so much, especially about living right and she always manage to tell what was right in love. Last but not least Bishop Harry L. Smith he was my spiritual father who supported me, mentored me and encouraged me when I was called to the ministry. I will always be thankful to you all and may God richly bless you!

Preface

Health and the health care industry have become major concerns in the United States for many years. During the twentieth century, we have seen an increase in health awareness and how essential it is for life. Everyone needs to attain some level of health because it is essential to how we function as humans and to live a life that is normal and enjoyable.

Consider the different health problems in this country. We are definitely in a health crisis, which is progressively getting worse. This country has seen a rise in many chronic and long-term physical and mental health problems. The numbers of people living with cardiovascular diseases, cancers, AIDS, and eating disorders have skyrocketed over the past fifty years. The mental and emotional damage of such long-term health problems has led to a society that is scrambling to address the country's health crisis.

Since 9/11 there has been an increase in the numbers of our military suffering from PTSD (post-traumatic stress disorder) because of war and other war-related injuries that have put a strain on our health care system, according to the Department of Veterans Affairs. This country proudly supports the war on terrorism, but we've had our military men and women come home without the ability to cope with life after multiple deployments, and now we have a serious problem. They come home with questions like how will I get treatment for my problems? Who will help me? What type of medical coverage will I be able to have?

When these soldiers are deployed, they are screened to see if they are fit for duty, but when they return home, they are screened to see if they are physically, mentally, and emotionally fit to return to normal life back home. This has led to an increase in domestic violence on many military installations, which in the past ten years has grown severe because service members have not gotten the preventive treatment they needed; nor do they receive adequate care and funding for their conditions. There is so much red tape and politics that confuses and frustrates many of our service members who have laid down their lives for this country. If this is happening to our own service members, imagine what is going on with people outside the military who can't afford health care.

People have needs, especially when it comes to health care and being able to afford it. Health care is a billion-dollar industry; so much money is used to fund all kinds of research for better medicine to handle certain health problems and conditions. When putting all of these issues into numbers, the statistics are astounding, especially the increase in the different types of health issues and the expenses for treatment that come with them. There are also the advertisements of many types of drugs that are being manufactured for some of these health conditions. Every day our society buys into this system to depend on these different types of medications for treatment which have been proven in some cases to be a cure, but the side effects of these medications are causing some serious issues. There have been many lawsuits, fines, and investigations because of these issues.

Is information made available by medical doctors on how to naturally lower your cholesterol? How to prevent another heart attack from occurring? There is always a push for more medication when in reality we can research and learn preventive measures to take better care of ourselves naturally. The statement heard many times that "an apple a day keeps the doctor away" is a true statement once you understand the concepts and the benefits of eating apples.

Most doctors won't tell you that there is a natural way to improve your health. They want to offer some type of drug because they're making a profit off the medications they prescribe. Why won't they tell you about other natural preventive measures? Makes you, ask what you are buying into as a society. I explain this statement in this book. There is a light at the end of the tunnel due to this health awareness. People are changing their way of living through an increase in the knowledge of health and being involved in healthy activities and knowing about good nutrition.

Health is not just only a physical problem; it's a spiritual problem as well. We focus so much on the physical, and we don't recognize that the spiritual is equally important in our lives. For example, looking at a person physically doesn't disclose that they have sound health, and it's equally important that looking at a person spiritually is the same. You don't know their spiritual condition.

Spiritual health is something that I believe most churches are not aware of, and there are people in our churches who can't heal spiritually because they aren't being fed the wholesome, healthy words of Jesus Christ. However, most churches are not being taught faith and how to believe for healing and simple restoration of the soul, which is where true healing begins. Most people in the church have been spiritually damaged by preachers whose teachings include a lot of error and have damaged many souls. In our churches, it has become a difficult task to heal these problems that are spiritual and physical. We have drowned out true believing that God heals through the work of faith in Jesus.

True healing comes from faith in the word of God, and this book will address many issues and critical questions about our spiritual health and development. If you see that this is important to you, take heed to how God can restore you spiritually by his grace and love. Think for a moment, what are the most important things in our lives that we value daily? Health is right there at the top of our list, I hope.

Our health is determined by the quality of living we choose for ourselves and our family. When you are searching for a place to live, you consider what the neighborhood is like and how the people live in that area. You evaluate the environment to see if it meets the standards that you want for your family. You determine the health and welfare of your family by your choices. You are careful in choosing where you want to raise your family and fostering a healthy environment for them to grow properly. The saying is true when looking for a place to live: "Location, location, location!" Location is very important. Health is a choice, and it's cultivated by changes in our lifestyle.

I encourage you to read this book with an open mind and heart to achieve success in every area of your life. Make sure as well that you are studying the word of God, which is more important. Jesus states it perfectly: "The thief cometh not, but for to steal, and to kill, and to destroy: I am come that they might have life, and that they might have it more abundantly" (John 10:10). We must work with a godly attitude to achieve the goal of spiritual health together.

The journey will be challenging, just as writing this book has been challenging for me, but it will be a good challenge for you to read and develop the mind-set to change your spiritual condition. The challenge also is that it begins with you and what you want out of life. Enjoy the journey that you are on with your Creator, who created all things available to you. He wants to restore us back to spiritual health, the way we were meant to be. I'm challenging you as a reader to be real with Jesus and show him that you mean business with him.

God wants us to live well, or he wouldn't have mentioned them in his word that he wants us to be blessed in every area of our lives. When I meet people, I always ask them the questions: How are you doing? How are you living? Are you living well? This is not just dealing with how you are living financially, though most people measure living well with what's in their bank account. There are a lot of wealthy people who are living a life of turmoil because money has become their god. They've developed an atmosphere where they are surrounded by toxic influences which have polluted and damaged their lives. We know that living in a polluted and toxic environment is unhealthy.

Unfortunately, for most of us, we're exposed to pollutants that can create serious health hazards. Spiritually speaking, we can suffer the same type of hazards if we don't take preventive measures to be aware of our spiritual surroundings. We are bombarded with a lot of garbage: toxic television shows, toxic people and influences of all kinds, toxic churches and their erroneous doctrines, and philosophies that are unscriptural. Remember the old nutrition statement that you heard for years: "You are what you eat." What you put inside you will promote either good health or bad health. The environment that you create will promote either good health or bad health.

My home life is a testimony that my wife and I have created in our home. Our daughters live in a healthy home because we chose the environment in which they can grow into healthy adults and become respectful and God-fearing women of character. Promoting a godly lifestyle is the hallmark and the foundation of the Christian life when it is operated based on faith in the word of God. Some of these lessons I had to learn the hard way because of my disobedience and the foolish mistakes that I've made that were damaging.

God is the only one who can transform a person's soul to peace and wholeness; this is one of his rich promises that we have when we obey his word. Second Timothy 1:7 says, "For God has not given us the spirit of fear; but of power, and of love, and of a sound mind." What stands out in that scripture is the *sound mind*, which means a mind that is healthy and at peace in God. When we learn to rely on the word of God, we benefit from faith in his word, and that faith activates the word of God, which means the word becomes life and has the ability to make us healthy. People in the world today are hurting and broken because society has overwhelmed them with a myriad of concerns and problems that affects their lives. What has happened spiritually is that we have amplified the troubles and problems of this world and minimized the effectiveness of God's word in our lives. We talk about our issues instead of seeing what God has to say about them.

He tells us to be at peace. Are you? He tells us not to let this world trouble us. Are you troubled? Remember, your faith is determined by how big is your God is. If you see God bigger than any of the circumstances that come into your life, then you have no worries. Remember in the movie *The Lion King*, the Swahili phrase *Hakuna Matata* can be translated literally as "no worries." God tells us not to worry. God's word is full of faith and power, and all you have to do is believe it and it will work for you. It is powerful enough to keep you from worrying if you have a working knowledge of it. Yes, we will be healed and whole, according to his word, so let's grow to be healthy, happy Christians!

So I want you to take your time. Thoroughly read this book, and look at it as a guide or a companion to the Bible. Because I have cited many passages of scripture to back up my text, so make sure that you are studying the Bible as well as build a basis for your understanding. I hope you enjoy the reading as I enjoyed writing this book, and may God bless you in your search for truth and understanding in the scriptures. May he bless you with peace, love, and happiness!

Introduction

On September 26, 2013, at 2:33 a.m., while I was in prayer, the Lord revealed to me the issue of the healing and health of the soul. I have a deep passion, compassion, and concern for people's lives and how they are living. When I start writing this book, I had in mind the idea that you will receive a wealth of information to show you that we can be healthy Christians and show people that there is a difference in the way we live. I have gained this information from a variety of sources, but most of them come from studying the word of God, personal experiences, and personal knowledge. My lovely wife told me to write it down and make it plain, and I thought to myself, sounds like the bible and sure enough, there was the scripture, Habakkuk 2:2–3 (NKJV):

> Then the LORD answered me and said: "Write the vision and make it plain on tablets, that he may run who reads it. For the vision is yet for an appointed time; But at the end it will speak, and it will not lie. Though it tarries, wait for it; because it will surely come, it will not tarry."

That inspired me! I wanted to write about things in my heart that I've learned for many years, things that I have a passion for. Now I want to make this clear, I'm not a doctor, a nutritionist, or some health specialist; nor am I some prolific author. I'm just an ordinary person like you with a passion for improving the quality of our living, and there's no greater way than to improve the way we live accept through faith in Jesus Christ. He's the focus and the source of our success in life. The scripture says, "Looking unto Jesus the author and the finisher of our faith" (Hebrews 12:2). So when I look for healing, health, life, and peace, Jesus is the answer for all of these things.

Our challenge is that we have to discover through his word the principles we need to apply to our lives. When I discuss later in the book about Jesus being our spiritual and natural physician, it means that he will heal the whole person with perfect soundness and wholeness. Christianity is not a religion; it's a way of life that is a direct relationship to a person, and that person is Jesus Christ. My passion for physical health, fitness, and nutrition has been a part of my life for many years. When I started writing, I began revealing to you, the reader, what God has given me, what I have experienced walking in the Word and how God has healed my soul to live a healthy life, both naturally and spiritually. I want you to experience the same joy that I have, allowing God to nourish you, and experiencing the true meaning of being healthy in the spirit.

God is a God of balance, and when we grasp God's laws of faith, we can exercise these principles to live a balanced life. We can't be so spiritual that we neglect the natural; neither can we be so natural that we neglect the spiritual. They both have to work together. For example, the word of God exhorts to walk in the spirit, and we will not fulfill the lust of the flesh—that's walking after the dictates of the flesh, which leads to sin and death (see Galatians 5:16–25). We must operate in these physical bodies by the Word of God, and it is the word that will dictate the way we should live. Taking care of your body, exercising, and staying active are not sins, and sometimes people think they add up to vanity. My question to those people is: What makes it vain?

Besides the body, the believer has a soul and a spirit; the first suggests the emotional and moral aspects of one's being, and the second entails the mental and spiritual part. Both of them need food. The emotional feeds on the great truths of the word which make God's love more real and precious and warm the heart; the spirit and intellect need to know the vital truths of scripture and to convey and teach them to others so that they may enlighten the mind.

We do not separate these two parts of man's spiritual makeup, but we do distinguish between them. Mere knowledge without the balance of emotional depth of a soul is apt to lead to pride (knowledge puffs up), and for this reason the believer is admonished to grow in grace and in the knowledge of our Lord and Savior, Jesus Christ—note, not merely the knowledge of him but to know him intimately. To know him is a great safeguard against the ever-possible exaltation of self. Likewise, emotional feeling without the corresponding knowledge of God's truth may lead to lack of wisdom and judgment and even to unbalanced fanaticism. The believer needs both a warm heart and a clear mind.

God wants us to be well on the inside as well as to look good on the outside. What we have that's on the inside will reflect what's on the outside. When God created man, he said that it was good, so God knew that he had created an incredible specimen. Look at it this way: if you are sick, weak, and unhealthy, how can you be a benefit to others? God wants us to be healed so we can, heal others physically, emotionally, and spiritually. What's wrong with looking nice? What's wrong with having a healthy appearance? What's wrong with having a muscular or an athletic physique? Absolutely nothing! It's all about a godly perspective based on the word of God, and that keeps it from becoming vain. When we learn to do things for the right reason we see that we can benefit and help others to achieve the joy of living healthy.

I like to keep things simple so that my life reflects simplicity. I try to exercise wisdom from the word of God, and this balances my life. Learning is a big part of my life, and I love to learn. For example, when I am learning from the word of God, my spirit is educated and nourished. There is a tremendous peace that fills my heart because

I have allowed the word of God to reside there. You can have all of these things; just be sure to stay humble and encourage and help people who want to be helped.

That brings up another issue. When it comes to wanting to be a help to others, some don't want to be helped, which to me is the denial of facing the truth about your issues. When we face the truth and embrace the truth, there is a release, and then there is relief, and it's wonderful. What does the scripture say? "And ye shall know the truth, and the truth shall make you free" (John 8:32). The word *is made* means to form (something) by putting parts together or combining substances; construct; create. This is saying that the words of Jesus will turn you into a person of freedom. We need to learn how to take good care of ourselves spiritually, physically, and emotionally.

One of the main focuses in the healing and health of the soul is look to Jesus as the one who will restore our souls, and when they are restored, they are healthy. He is the soul doctor to all humanity, and his desire is to restore you back to the way God intended for you to live.

Take a look at the scripture in Luke 4:18: "The Spirit of the Lord is upon me, because he has anointed me to preach the gospel to the poor; he hath sent me to heal the brokenhearted, to preach deliverance to the captives, and recovering of sight to the blind, to set at liberty them that are bruised...." This passage of scripture is about healing and restoration, and most of Jesus' ministry was about healing. Health is not something that happens overnight; it takes time and patience, the same way it is spiritually: you develop that peace in your spirit over time, and it takes effort in wanting to seek God's word for that peace and wholeness in your spirit. All of us were not healed overnight; it took some time, medication, and someone who genuinely cared about our recovery or our restoration. Jesus is our physical therapist to bring about true healing in the hearts and minds of his people.

If you get down to the root of every issue in people's lives, you will find out that the cause is something spiritual. When we were born into this world, we were subject to the pollutions of this world because of the fall of man. Not only does Jesus want to restore us, he wants to bring order back into our lives, and he does it by grace and faith in his Word. I will quote this saying a lot about the richness of God's word in your spirit, and you will not have lack in your life when you act on what's been put in you. The word of God is your foundation for life, and I want you to experience the best that God has for you.

Remember that my only intention is to be concerned about the lives of people who have been damaged spiritually and physically. Lives are at stake here, and it's imperative that we learn by biblical truth how to restore people's lives by the word. The restoration of the human race is a work only God can do. Our part is to be obedient to the word of God, and he will show us his goodness and guide us in the right things to do for others.

God not only wants to restore us, but he will one day restore this earth to its rightful state spiritually and naturally. We believe that Jesus is coming; through his righteous judgment, he will renovate this earth and make it new again. The scripture states it this way in the book of Romans: "We know that the whole creation has been groaning as in the pains of childbirth right up to the present time. Not only so, but we ourselves, who have the first fruits of the Spirit, groan inwardly as we wait eagerly for our adoption to sonship, the redemption of our bodies" (Romans 8:22–23 NIV). This lets us know that even creation is groaning for restoration. You can see things happening every day, making it clear that something is wrong with this world. This world is polluted with toxins and chemicals, causing us to have all kinds of health problems. Unusual incidents involve animals, such as thousands of whales showing up dead on a seashore; animal diseases that sweep the country, killing a lot of our livestock; and the many different cases of harmful bacteria that attack our crops, which produce most of the food we eat. Many food products and goods we buy have had to be recalled due to widespread fears of contamination.

All these severe problems, issues, and destruction is why I know Jesus Christ must come back to restore this earth. We're making a conscious effort to come up with legislation to preserve our natural resources and animals that are considered to be endangered species, and we have accomplished a lot. But this doesn't scratch the surface because this is a global problem that only God himself can handle. So for our part, we look for a new heaven and earth, and this is the promise that God made in his word according to 2 Peter 3:13. Restoration, peace, and happiness are coming to this earth, and King Jesus is bringing them with him. So trust in the Lord for restoration for your soul, because according to Malachi 4:2 he is coming with healing in his wings.

1

WHAT IS HEALTH?

Beloved, I wish above all things that thou may prosper
and be in health, even as thy soul prospered.

—3 John 2

My son, give attention to my words;
Incline your ear to my sayings.
Do not let them depart from your eyes;
Keep them in the midst of your heart;
For they *are* life to those who find them,
And health to all their flesh.

—Proverbs 4:20–22 (NKJV)

Question: What does it mean to be healthy and whole? What
does the word *healthy* mean for you? Let's make this personal—are
you healthy spiritually? We will dig deeply into the spiritual meaning
of the word *health, according* to the scriptures, and we will find out
what the word of God has to say about our spiritual health.

Before we can understand and comprehend the spiritual
meaning, let's take a look at the natural meaning of the word *health.*
Jesus always used a parable, which is a short allegorical story used to
illustrate a spiritual principle or concept so that the lesson taught can

1

be understood and made clear to the hearers of the story. With that said, let's look at the natural definition of the word *health* to grasp the natural concept of health before we transition to the spiritual concept of health. This greatly enhances our understanding of how essential both physical and spiritual health is to the overall health of a person's body, mind, and spirit. So what is healthy in its natural sense of the word? Let's take a look.

Health is the level of functional or metabolic efficiency of a living organism. In humans, it is the general condition of a person's mind and body, and it usually connotes being free from illness, injury, or pain (as in "good health" or "health"). The World Health Organization (WHO) defined health in its broader sense in 1946 as "a state of complete physical, mental, and social well-being and not merely the absence of disease or infirmity." The term *healthy* is also widely used in the context of many types of nonliving organizations and their effects for the benefit of humans, as in the sense of healthy communities, healthy cities, or healthy environments. In addition to health care interventions and a person's surroundings, a number of other factors are known to influence the health status of individuals, including their backgrounds, lifestyles, and economic and social conditions; these are referred to as "determinants of health."

Generally, the context in which an individual lives is of great importance for his or her health status and quality of life. It is increasingly recognized that health is maintained and improved not only through the advancement and application of health science, but also through the efforts and intelligent lifestyle choices of the individual and society. According to the World Health Organization, the main determinants of health include the social and economic environment, the physical environment, and the person's individual characteristics and behaviors.

Many choices that we make in life have an impact on how we live our lives and how healthy we are. Every day we make choices, and they will lead either to rewards and benefits or to trouble and consequences—the choice is ours. Joshua 24:15 states: "And if it seem evil unto you to serve the LORD, choose you this day whom ye will serve; whether the gods which your fathers served that were on the other side of the flood, or the gods of the Amorites, in whose land I dwell: but as for me and my house, we will serve the LORD." In other words, we choose how we want to live our lives.

God will always allow us to make choices, even if they hurt us; this sounds harsh, but it is a reality of life. We must realize as believers that God is the only one who can heal us and restore us after we have made bad decisions. I know, and I am living proof of that spiritual restoration; I am now experiencing what it's like being spiritually healthy.

Being a fitness enthusiast and mentor in the military, I became more concerned for others' health and wanted to help them develop healthy habits that promote a healthy and enjoyable lifestyle. I have frequently counseled individuals, and the first thing that they notice is that they feel better in general and about their accomplishments; there is a rejuvenated awareness that they feel and that's important when you begin to improve your health. This isn't talking about how big you want your biceps to be or how much you can bench or how big you want to be. I have heard that kind of gym jargon a lot, especially when I'm deployed. All these soldiers come up with unrealistic goals about what they are going to do when they get in the gym. Don't adopt that philosophy. Here is the question: Are you healthy inside? Have you heard of internal health? Is your organs functioning properly? We are still dealing with the natural part of us that is essential for God to use us for his service. Stick with me; I am going somewhere with this subject. This is health talk 101.

We must understand the concept of being healthy spiritually and naturally and there must also be balance in our philosophy about both. Read this statement: "Achieving and maintaining health is an ongoing process shaped by both the evolution of healthcare knowledge and practices and personal strategies and organized interventions for staying healthy—known as lifestyle management." To add to that statement, you must put in some effort to acquire the resources to improve your health. If you want to be helped, you will find the resources to help you achieve that goal. When you start taking charge in managing your life in your health, finances, and family, you will gain more rewards than you can imagine.

Developing yourself is determined by the resources you acquire and apply to improve your health and life, and doing this will make you a valuable asset to yourself, your family, and others who need you. When you think about health, think of your family. Think of what it will be like if you take better care of yourself, and think about what it will be like when you improve yourself. What I get out of it is how I feel because I looked for the help and counseling to improve my life. I have a lovely wife and two beautiful girls, and they need me every day. It's a personal endeavor of mine to stay healthy and be consistent with my healthy habits, which have benefited me for many years.

I want to share a personal testimony about my health prior to being deployed in 2011. I was always very conscious of my physical health and fitness. Being in the military for more than twenty-eight years, meeting those requirements to stay healthy and fit is one of the most important achievements if I wanted to stay in the military. During the pre-deployment process, we were screened to see if we were fit for duty. After the results came back, they said that my cholesterol and my blood pressure were high enough to cause concern. The doctor's suggestion was to put me on medication, and I wasn't ready to accept being on some type of drug for the rest of my life. This motivated me to do something about it, so I began to research natural ways to lower blood pressure and cholesterol. I looked into the benefits of drinking green tea, eating certain raw fruits and vegetables, and taking good, healthy supplements. Then of course I exercised religiously six times a week, and I controlled what I ate each day.

You see something here? This is an example of personal management and taking personal responsibility for your life. Also, I continued to look for more ways to enhance my fitness through study and research. After about two months applying what I had learned, the results were amazing; I dropped my cholesterol and my blood pressure down to their normal ranges, and I dropped my body fat from 22 percent down to 12 percent. Remember, achieving and maintaining your health is an ongoing process. I didn't just eat something healthy once and expect to see the benefits in one day; it took some time, motivation, and discipline to achieve that goal, but it is extremely rewarding when you achieve it.

Basically, I improved my health and overall fitness. I put forth the effort, did research, and talked to people who know this stuff. You should always ask questions about your condition before you start taking drugs that can lead to all kinds of problems in your body. You think that most of these doctors are there to make you well, but I've heard horror stories about patients getting worse due to the drugs, which have caused severe side effects. Some of the side effects can be downright fatal, causing millions of dollars in lawsuits because of malpractice in the medical field.

I'm saying don't just listen to your doctors about the medications they prescribe for you. Medicine is needful, or else God would not have given humans the ability to practice and find out what the body needs for wellness. You can prevent a lot of this nonsense by taking the wise approach in your health, and many of your answers are just a keystroke away. Please don't get me wrong, doctors are helpful, and they are very important in finding out what's wrong with us; some of them do an impeccable job of diagnosing what's the cause in our bodies. They are needful and rightfully so, and I thank God for them, and many of them have an impeccable reputation for what they do. Please see your doctor on a regular basis; it is essential for knowing the status of your health.

While improving your health with effort on your part you can probably wean yourself off from some of these drugs. Case in point, your liver actually processes all of these drugs, and some cases that I've heard have led to severe liver damage and even death. Remember phen-phen? This supplement killed people, and many lawsuits were the result. I personally know of a friend of mine who lost his wife due to this product. Yes, he received a large amount of money in settlement, but at a price that's tragic.

Spend some time finding out about yourself physically, mentally, and spiritually; what you discover will surprise you. For example, I thought I had this health stuffed figured out, and I was wrong! Once you find out what you can do about it—and you have the power to do something about it—then it becomes a motivating force to accomplish and achieve your goals. Believe me when I tell you this, once you experience results, you will become intrigued, and you will build on what you have learned. This is the exciting part: nutrition, exercise, and the continuing journey of discovery together becomes a way of life, and a lot of your health issues can be solved.

Remember, the key to all of this is time, and time is of the essence to optimal health. It's often said that "time heals all wounds." Yes, that's true, but you have to have the right resources and surround yourself with the right people for those wounds to heal properly. Without the proper context, time will not heal all wounds, and many times they are suppressed and are never dealt with in the quest for true healing. We are on our way to spiritual health, and this just the beginning of it. We will take time and build together the concept of being healthy, healed, and whole in body, mind, and spirit. I want you to be blessed in discovering what God wants you to be.

God is interested in the total person, and he wants you to be fully interested in him. Jesus states it this way: "Thou shall love the Lord thy God with all thy heart, and with all thy soul, and with all thy strength, and with the entire mind" (Luke 10:27). Look at that heart and soul of a person; that's what God wants, and he wants to make use of you for his glory. God wants us to always present ourselves to him for service, so we have to be healthy for the service. Romans 12:1 says, "I beseech you therefore, brethren, by the mercies of God, that ye present your bodies a living sacrifice, holy, acceptable unto God, which is your reasonable service." We are representatives of the Lord, and we have to represent him in everything we do. In the military when we show up for duty, we are expected to be in the right uniform and well groomed for the day's duty and it's a part of the military life. The military calls its readiness for service, and that is the concept I draw from this scripture: God wants us to be spiritually, physically and emotionally ready to serve him.

How are you being a representative for him? What is it about the way you live that causes people either to be attracted to you or to want not to be around you? This takes some soul and heart searching to see where we fit in that statement. Our lives are being watched, and we need to show others a healthy lifestyle. Physical health is a wonderful blessing, but health of soul and spirit is far more to be desired, not only for its own sake, but also because it is a mighty contributing factor in robust, physical well-being.

What's going on inside of a person as far as their health is concerned? Hold that thought. In chapter 1 we have discussed the meaning of health and looked at the importance of why our health is essential to our daily lives. We discussed why choosing a better way to live will have lasting benefits on how we live. Every day, adopt new ways of doing things that will promote health and one of those is to look at what is going on in your physical body.

When we deal with people on a regular basis on the job and in our churches, schools, and communities, we have relationships with people about whom we really know very little unless we begin to sit down, have conversations with each other, and develop healthy relationships. What's interesting is that you find out a lot about a person when you start talking, whether good, bad, or indifferent. People in general are interesting; yes, some are weird or "crazy," and some have odd personalities. That's okay because we are all unique in a special way.

Sometimes you just don't know who you are talking to, and the scripture even relates that some of us have entertained angels and are unaware of it. This is what the word of God has to say in Hebrews 13:2: "Be not forgetful to entertain strangers: for thereby some have entertained angels unawares." My point is you never know who you are talking to, what they are going through, and what is going on in their mind.

Sometimes we use the statement "perception is everything," but are you sure? We can perceive something in a certain way, and that leads to making an assumption, and most of the time we are wrong because we don't know the whole story about a person. The word of God is right when it says that out of the abundance of the heart the mouth will speak. As we spend time around people, they will speak, and it may not be pleasant sometimes, so get ready. Don't be surprised what comes out of people. Because they are telling a story of an internal struggle, pay attention and weigh their words, and you will find out what they really mean by their words.

That's why I love the Lord Jesus: he knows the whole story, and he will let me plead my case without any interruptions. He will let me speak what's on my mind because he knows me better than anybody. He knows what's going on inside, and he is there to heal whatever is troubling my spirit.

God heals your spirit, and then it manifests in the natural. The root cause to almost every human issue is usually something spiritual. We tend to look at the psychological aspect of the situation, sensing that something beyond the natural might be causing the problem.

There is an external health that we display, and we assume that we are healthy based on our outward appearance. Looks can be very deceiving. We know that a person can look perfectly all right and not know that they are deteriorating inside. Sometimes people have a troubled or disturbed mind, and you don't know until they snap or you take notice of their behavior patterns. You've heard many of the classic statements about a person after the damage is done:

- He looked perfectly all right to me.
- I didn't know she had a heart problem.
- We didn't see the signs, or we weren't aware of the signs.

This is just to name a few. I didn't get into mental health, an issue that's become a widespread problem in our society today. Physicians and specialists are professionals, trained to be able to look at our bodies through tests and studies to diagnose what can be causing a sickness, injury, or ailment in the body. There are several ways they can run tests to see what is going on, and we who have been in the hospital know that they will take samples of fluid from your body; usually it consists of a blood or urine sample. They know that if there is an infection in the body, there will be an increase in white blood cell count because white blood cells are designed to fight infections.

Whatever happens in the body, it's usually detected either in the urine or blood. This is what the word of God has to say: "The life of every creature is its blood. That is why I have said to the Israelites, 'you must not eat the blood of any creature, because the life of every creature is its blood; anyone who eats it must be cut off'" (Leviticus 17:14 NIV). God knows the activity, and whatever is going on, it's in that blood. Based on medical procedures, doctors have to have these tests done so they can accurately diagnose the problem and administer the correct treatment to make the individual well. We are stewards (managers) of our own bodies, and we are responsible for how we control them.

Internal health means every organ in the body is functioning normally. This is achieved through internal medicine and nutrition, and the process of healing is the result. When there is internal healing, there are wellness and relief in the body.

Healing is a process, often involving medical, surgical, or psychiatric treatment of a pathological condition, which culminates in the functional repair, and sometimes the actual regeneration, of a previously diseased or damaged part of the body or mind. That's why therapy must be addressed to parts of the body that have been injured or damaged.

I want to share another testimony about healing as a process and why we need assistance in getting that healing properly. When I was deployed several years ago, I began to experience back pain

9

from wearing body armor. I tried everything, stretching out my back at night before I went to bed. Sometimes I would have my wife to try to pop my back, and she would step on it, which sometimes brought temporarily relief. I tried everything except the right thing, and that was going to see a chiropractor to find out what was really the problem—what caused my back to have so much pain and what was the source.

After taking some x-rays, he noticed that in the middle of my back there was a small curvature which had a misalignment which was causing the pain. He said that over a period of time, several things could cause my back to be in so much pain. One was obviously the body armor, which caused my spine to be compressed over a period of time, the mattress that I was sleeping on, and of course the day-to-day activities of life. He showed me the different types of treatments that they might perform. He said that a single visit would not fix the problem. His idea of treatment involved a period of time, but even after the first treatment I felt great relief.

I just want to interject a thought here for a moment: sometimes we can get a temporary fix to a long-term problem and we feel that we are all right. But we still haven't fixed the source, and that is where we go wrong when we are being helped. We fail to get to the root of the health issue. We need to dig deep into the source of the issue to find out how to heal properly. You don't put a Band-Aid on a broken arm; it's the wrong treatment! You find out the problem, and over time, with the right treatment, you can advance the healing process the right way.

That was what happened to me. Week after week I went to the chiropractor for treatments, and over a period of time my back condition improved. The chiropractor also took another set of x-rays a few months later, and I had a healthy-looking spine. The key to my healing was the right doctor, the right diagnosis, the right treatment, and time; this is the healing process. This caused my back to heal the right way.

We must make sure that we are serious when dealing with our

health whether it's physical or spiritual. We must make sure that the right people are involved in our healing process. Not everybody knows how to heal; that's why, when going to a doctor, you make sure that you go to the specific doctor for your health issue. Sometimes for healing and achieving good health you have to be honest with yourself about any health issue that you have. Don't be in denial that there is a problem; part of the healing is admitting the problem to yourself, not to other people.

Health is a way of life, and you are the one who will determine your level of health based on your own discipline and desires. Remember that health is physical, mental, emotional, and spiritual, and they are all important to a person's whole being. When you start practicing good, healthy habits and staying involved in healthy activities daily, you will have a very good perspective on life. Your attitude will determine that.

The word of God is absolutely the best place to start; it has an amazing effect on your physical health, and when the word is believed, it can bring healing and health to our bodies. The word of God has the ability to penetrate into any damaged soul, find the problem, and heal it with grace and power.

God wants every part of our life to be well-balanced, because sometimes we can go to an extreme with anything, and we can ruin our lives when we do not have wisdom in the things we do. For example, we should exercise, but we can take it to extremes and injure ourselves without the proper understanding of nutrition, exercise, and rest. If you take a look at nature, you can see that God is a God of balance, and it is his desire for us to be the same way. People have their own opinions about eating: one might say you should eat nothing but fruits and vegetables, while another would say you should eat meat. Perhaps you need them both, but in moderation. For example, you need meat or some source of protein for muscle building, and some meats are high in iron (red meat like steaks), but you shouldn't eat too much of it. You need vegetables such as carrots, which are good for the eyes because they contain a nutrient called beta-carotene, a substance that the body converts to vitamin A, an important nutrient for eye health. You need fruits such as grapefruit, which actually burns fat around the organs. It also has a powerful nutrient called pectin, also found in apples, which can help lower cholesterol and lower your blood pressure.

So you see, you need a variety of all foods for overall nourishment of the body. Think of a car; what are the fluids that a car needs to function properly? It needs fuel, oil, transmission fluid, water, and antifreeze because of the different mechanical functions of the car. All these fluids work differently and are designed for different purposes. You don't put antifreeze into the gas tank; nor do you put water in the engine.

It's the same way with your body: you need a variety of all kinds of foods to get a complete supply of nutrients for the normal functions of the body. Specific foods are needed for specific functions of the body. Feeding your body protein is essential for muscle building and repair; that's specifically what it is designed for.

God's word is the same way it has spiritual building ingredients that are essential for making your spirit robust. One thing that I experienced is that the Word of God is designed and tailored to fit everybody's needs. God is very specific in wanting you to know how to handle different situations in your life. What I mean is that when you are dealing with different situations, you need to feed your spirit a specific utterance of the word of God for that problem. I've learned through this the idea of keeping things simple; don't be confused and enslave yourself to what you can or can't eat. Get the knowledge and understanding, and you will have the freedom to eat and enjoy it. This understanding about health is not to put you under a strict program to keep you from enjoying life. Remember, God gives us all things to enjoy.

My intention is for you to be aware of the benefits as well as the consequences for the condition of your health. Your health physically and spiritually is the hallmark of your life. It is the foundation of wellness to the body and soul. When an individual is healthy in body and soul, it will be seen in that person's life. Later in the book I will be discussing how to enjoy life—for example, laughter, and I mean a good, loud, gut-wrenching laugh, which is what I do often. It really doesn't take much for me to laugh; it's wonderful, and I enjoy it. I don't want to get ahead of myself about what I want to discuss in this, because there is a lot about being able to enjoy life God's way. I am excited in my spirit to discuss what I have learned through the knowledge of the word of God and how I have practiced these concepts for many years, and I tell you that they work. They produce not just a healthy life, but a life of holiness. As my father-in-law says, just living right is healthy because you set the spiritual thermostat in your home when you are living a healthy, clean life before the Lord. I wouldn't want it any other way. This is a true statement that the word of God will make you if you allow it to make you. God is not going to force you to be healthy, neither is anybody who is motivated to helping you. In his third Epistle, John said I wish that you will prosper and be in good health (verse 2); he never made it a command. My point is that I think that we will miss out on the blessings and benefits if we don't seek health and prosperity. We just need to keep it in the right perspective which is based on kingdom principles from the word of God.

Jesus is the chief builder of the church. Like a shepherd, he takes care of his sheep, and he protects and defends the sheep. More importantly, he feeds his sheep the wholesome words from his mouth. The scripture says: "All bare Him witness, and wondered at the gracious words which proceeded out of his mouth" (Luke 4:22). Just as your physical health will decline if you don't continue to practice healthy habits and feed your body good nutrition, so it is with your spiritual health: you will deteriorate if you decide to depart from the teachings of the Lord Jesus. With no guidance and stability, you have no way to stay on track spiritually with God's direction.

I'd like to challenge the reader of this book, whether you are a believer or not to these statements: If there is anybody out there who can say that they have a better way of living than the life that

God offers, I would like them to let me know. I'm an open-minded person, and I'd like to be educated and corrected as necessary if I'm wrong. Let me know if you have something to offer that is better than the Lord Jesus. Do you think you will be able to convince me? My first question would be, can you offer me peace of mind? Can you offer rest to my soul? Can you heal me? There is nobody on this earth qualified to do this but Jesus alone.

The great news about all of this that when he invites all who are weary and burdened to "come unto me," he means everybody (see Matthew 11:28–30). Just as you have a choice whether to live a healthy life, so it is with God: you have a choice to make him Lord and Savior of your life. Christ is able to manage every aspect of your life with grace, mercy, and love that the world cannot offer. I challenge you to pursue the life of God through our Lord Jesus and watch him restore, heal, and bring peace to your soul. You will experience an abundance of grace in your life that can't be explained. It's just awesome how he wants to make your soul healthy!

2

WHAT IS NUTRITION?

If thou put the brethren in remembrance of these things, thou shall be a good minister of Jesus Christ, nourished up in the words of faith and of good doctrine, whereunto thou hast attained.

—1 Timothy 4:6

Nutrition is a major factor of a healthy body, and what you put into your body greatly affects the way your body performs. When the body is not performing well, it's usually a nutritional deficiency that causes the problem; we call this malnourishment or malnutrition. When I began to study nutrition, I was intrigued with how food works in the body and what benefits you get out of good, nutritious foods. Spiritual nutrition works the same; you become what you feed your spirit every day. When you feed your body good, nutritious meals, your body will be nourished with essential vitamins and minerals for it to perform well.

Likewise, when you feed your mind and heart the word of God by faith, your spirit will reap the benefits of faith in that word. When you feed your mind the wrong things, like erroneous, toxic teachings, you pollute your soul, damaging its health, and the effects are detrimental. You become a product of that teaching; you develop wrong thinking and justify behavior that is out of line with the word of God; that's the ultimate effect of bad teaching. On the positive side, when you feed your soul the word of God, by faith you develop the right concept of doing things God's way. Believers who go through trials and tribulations and are not shaken by the problems are so filled with nourishment of the word of God that they handle the problems with confidence.

That's what happens when you feed your mind the word of God. As Kenneth Hagin states it, "The word of God is faith food for the soul." Another famous preacher has said that "when you feed your faith, you will starve your doubts to death." We will get into the spiritual side later; I just needed to add some essential true statements to enhance our understanding about what we are putting into our bodies physically and spiritually. I want you to understand the natural so you can grasp the spiritual concept later. The statement is true, as I said earlier, that "you are what you eat." Now don't get me wrong. I'm not a health nut; I eat junk foods occasionally; and I enjoy them when I eat them. But if you develop a discipline in your eating habits, one junk food meal will not bother you at all because you have developed a healthy eating habit that's improving your health and promoting a healthy lifestyle.

Quotes to live by about nutrition:

"Let food be your medicine and medicine be your food." (Hippocrates)

"The doctor of the future will give no medicines, but will interest his patients in the care of the human frame, in diet, and in the cause and prevention of disease." (Thomas Edison)

"He who has health has hope, and he who has hope has everything." (Arabian Proverb)

"He that takes medicine and neglects diet wastes the skills of the physician." (Chinese proverb)

What is nutrition? Simply said, nutrition is the study of food at work in our bodies, our source for energy, and the medium for which our nutrients can function. Think of nutrition as the building blocks of life. The essential nutrients for life include carbohydrates, proteins, and lipids (fats), as well as fiber, vitamins, minerals, and water—the solvent for all soluble ingredients in the blood and cells. The absorption of nutrients starts the moment we begin to digest our foods, as they are transported to assist all the metabolic processes in the human body.

Good nutrition means getting the right amount of nutrients from healthy foods in the right combinations. Having nutrition knowledge and making smart choices about the foods you eat can and will help you achieve optimum health over your lifetime and is a key to avoiding obesity, illness, and many of today's most prevalent chronic diseases. Nutrition is just one key to developing and maintaining good health. Good health is defined as a state of complete physical, mental, and social well-being—a healthy mind, body, and spirit. Nutrition is at work during our entire life-cycle— from infancy to adolescence and into adulthood and through our senior years—and can be the antidote for many of today's common problems, such as stress, pollution, sexual dysfunction, and disease.

For me personally, nutrition translates into health, and health is freedom. Being healthy not only makes us feel great, it enables us to enjoy life to our fullest potential, and to follow our dreams. Conversely, a poor diet can have a serious impact on health, and rob you of your freedom. Food therapy is emerging as the latest prevention against multiple lifestyle diseases. Experts now believe that popping an apple is better than popping a pill. Negative influences such as stress, shock, injury, emotional upsets, and worries can have a direct impact on lifelong health. The good news is that the body can heal itself, if given what it needs to do its job. The nutrition in certain foods can naturally increase your body's oxygen levels, eliminate many sources of toxins, improve your digestion, and prevent, heal, or reduce the severity of various diseases.

Nutrition is about choices. Healthy eating is the best recipe for an abundant life. Make every bite count. You don't have to get very picky when it comes to eating healthy, and don't put yourself under stress when it comes to food choices. Some people count every calorie and rob themselves of the ability to enjoy food. I like to always think simple and be practical in my approach when it comes to healthy eating. When you begin to practice this healthy lifestyle, it will set you apart from sedentary people who don't practice these things at all. Your way of life, how you look at life, your attitude, and your perspective about issues will be different. You'll approach life with confidence, and you will have a certain mind-set because you have made this a way of life for yourself.

When you look into the word of God, you see many examples of the way God wants us to live. In the Old Testament, when God delivered Israel from Egypt, he had a purpose for them: he wanted his people to be different for his divine purpose. One of those differences was their diet—they had strict guidelines on what to eat and what not to eat, and it was to show their devotion to the Lord. God knows about health better than we do; he created all the healthy foods and wants us to discover all the things that he has for us to enjoy. He wants us to enjoy life and to have balance in our lives physically and spiritually. He wants us to have control and discipline in how we behave daily. We are accountable to him, so he expects us to live a certain way and to be different from the world.

Do you remember the word *sedentary*? Some people are physically sedentary, and some are spiritually sedentary. This fact is observable everywhere. There are people who have no drive to do anything, and their life is ordinary: there's no life in them, and they just go through life aimlessly without any purpose or drive to do anything. Spiritually, there are people who go to church, and that's all they do. They are not actively involved in their own spiritual development in faith, in the word of God on a daily basis.

What in the world is sedentary? A sedentary lifestyle is a type of lifestyle with irregular physical activity or little or none. A person who lives a sedentary lifestyle is what we may colloquially call a couch potato. The condition is commonly found in both the developed and developing worlds. Sedentary activities include sitting, reading, watching television, playing video games, and computer use for much of the day with little or no vigorous physical exercise.

A sedentary lifestyle can contribute to many preventable causes of death. Screen time is the amount of time a person spends watching a screen such as a television, computer monitor, or mobile device. Excessive screen time is linked to negative health consequences. A lack of physical activity is one of the leading causes of preventable death worldwide.

Sitting still may cause premature death. The risk is higher among those who sit still more than five hours per day. It is shown to be a risk factor on its own, independent of hard exercise and BMI (body mass index), which correlates to risk of chronic diseases. People who sit still more than four hours per day have a 40 percent higher risk than those who sit less than four hours per day. However, people who exercise at least four hours per week are as healthy as those who sit less than four hours per day.

Sedentary lifestyle and lack of physical activity can contribute to or be a risk factor for:

- Anxiety
- Cardiovascular disease
- Mortality in elderly men (increased by 30 percent; risk is doubled in elderly women)
- Deep vein thrombosis
- Depression
- Diabetes
- Colon cancer
- High blood pressure
- Obesity

- Osteoporosis
- Lipid disorders
- Kidney stones

These health risk factors can be reduced through effort on our part. For example, a machine needs periodic maintenance against wear and tear. That's why you need mechanics and other maintenance personnel. It's the same way with your body: it needs be maintained through regular exercise and good nutrition to perform well. If you don't maintain it properly, it will not perform properly, just as with a machine.

When I think of the word *nutrition*, I think of other words related to it like *nourishing, wholesome*, and *fortified*. These words are associated with healthy eating to ensure that the body is receiving the right nutrition. What's going on in the body when you eat or drink? It's something that we don't often think about until it is too late, when the damage is already done.

Let's look at some foods and drinks that are simple just to get an idea about how food affects the body. We know water is essential to life on planet Earth. We need to drink a lot of it because of the many benefits it provides. These are some of the benefits of drinking water:

- Hydrates the body and prevents it from overheating.
- Detoxifies the body by ridding it of toxins, which reduces kidney stones and helps stop ailments like headaches and constipation.
- Improves skin tone and clears up dry skin, causing you to have a youthful appearance.
- Improves function of the liver, the main organ used to metabolize proteins, carbohydrates, and fats. The liver is the body's processes, and an adequate water supply daily, will promote the loss of weight. It will also stimulate liver function to burn more body fat, which essential to weight loss.

There are a wide variety of fruits and vegetables to choose from that we need to improve our health. For example, eating apples will improve your health and overall wellness in many ways. Here are some of the benefits of eating apples:

- Reduce cholesterol. The soluble fiber found in apples binds with fats in the intestine, which translates into lower cholesterol levels and a healthier you.
- Help stabilize blood sugar to decrease your risk of diabetes.
- Get a healthier heart. The phenolic compound found in apple skins also prevents the cholesterol that gets into your system from solidifying on your artery walls. When plaque builds inside your arteries, it reduces blood flow to your heart, leading to coronary artery disease.
- Beat diarrhea and constipation. Whether you can't go to the bathroom or you just can't stop, the fiber found in apples can help. Fiber can either pull water into your colon to keep things moving along when you're backed up, or absorb excess water from your stool to slow your bowels down.
- Neutralize irritable bowel syndrome. Irritable bowel syndrome is characterized by constipation, diarrhea, and abdominal pain and bloating. To control these symptoms, doctors recommend staying away from dairy and fatty foods while including a high intake of fiber in your diet.
- Control your weight. Apples will curb your appetite so you will not snack on unhealthy foods and cause weight gain. To manage your weight and improve your overall health, doctors recommend a diet rich in fiber. Foods high in fiber will fill you up without costing you too many calories.
- Detoxify your liver. We're constantly consuming toxins, whether it is from drinks or food, and your liver is responsible for clearing these toxins out of your body. Many doctors are skeptical of fad detox diets, saying they have the potential to do more harm than good. Luckily, one of the best and

easiest things you can eat to help detoxify your liver is fruits like apples.

- Boost your immune system. Red apples contain an antioxidant called quercetin. Recent studies have found that quercetin can help boost and fortify your immune system, especially when you're stressed out.
- Apples contain a plethora of phytochemicals called flavonoids. These flavonoids have a major role as antioxidants. The health benefits of these antioxidants include curing stomach disorders in infants, resolving constipation and diarrhea in babies, curing a cough, and aiding dental disorders in babies.

Let take a look at one more measure that I have found playing an important role in my weight reduction, and that's drinking green tea. Green tea has powerful antioxidants and phenols used to promote lowering of cholesterol and high blood pressure. They also help in the prevention of many types of cancers and sickness.

These are just examples of a few foods that can improve your health over a period of time. Never once did I mention any type of drug; good nutrition is your drug for optimal performance, health, and wellness to the human body. We know how essential it is for us to stay healthy for God's service, to do his will on the earth. The military uses the expression "fit for duty," and you often hear the saying "fit for life." We need to be fit for God's service, and we need to represent him in a way that is pleasing to him in our way of life.

The book of Daniel gives a good illustration about being different and not living a sedentary lifestyle Daniel 1:1–20. Here we read about Nebuchadnezzar, king of Babylon, who came to Jerusalem, besieged the nation of Israel, and carried them back to Babylon. King Nebuchadnezzar ruled over Israel and demanded that they learn the language and literature of the Babylonians. Certain men were chosen from the children of Israel who were skilled in all kinds of craft, wisdom, and knowledge that could benefit the king's kingdom.

Daniel, Shadrach, Meshach, and Abednego were among those chosen for this task. King Nebuchadnezzar wanted to indoctrinate them into the Babylonian lifestyle, particularly their diet.

Daniel, who believed in God (Jehovah), didn't forget the Mosaic commandments of the law, not to defile himself with the diet of the Babylonians. Daniel purposed in his heart not to eat their food, and he asked his chief official for permission not to defile himself this way. This request went totally against the king's wishes, so God caused the official to show favor and compassion to Daniel and his friends. Daniel asked a favor of the chief official that instead of making the four of them eat the king's food, they should receive vegetables and water to drink for ten days. Then the official could judge whether they were healthier than the Babylonians. Let's look at this word for word according to the scriptures to see the outcome of this story.

> [Daniel said to their guard assigned by the official] "Please test your servants for ten days: Give us nothing but vegetables to eat and water to drink. Then compare our appearance with that of the young men who eat the royal food, and treat your servants in accordance with what you see." So he agreed to this and tested them for ten days.

> At the end of the ten days they looked healthier and better nourished than any of the young men who ate the royal food. So the guard took away their choice food and the wine they were to drink and gave them vegetables instead. (Daniel 1:12–16 NIV)

The lesson in the story was that when the chief official saw that they had a healthier appearance than the others, he was impressed and gave them more of the same. So he saw the results and the benefits of eating healthy foods.

Let look at what the king had to say when they had to present themselves to the king.

> To these four young men God gave knowledge and understanding of all kinds of literature and learning. And Daniel could understand visions and dreams of all kinds.
>
> At the end of the time set by the king to bring them into his service, the chief official presented them to Nebuchadnezzar. The king talked with them, and he found none equal to Daniel, Shadrach, Meshach, and Abednego; so they entered the king's service. In every matter of wisdom and understanding about which the king questioned them, he found them ten times better than all the magicians and enchanters in his whole kingdom. (Daniel 1:17–20 NIV)

They don't seem sedentary to me; they chose and purposed in their heart not be like the others but declared that they would be different. What made the difference was that God was with them and honored them, so he blessed them under the captivity and rule of King Nebuchadnezzar. Daniel was confident in his convictions to be different and not settle for the king's type of lifestyle, even though he was in captivity. Daniel didn't settle for the ordinary; he achieved the extraordinary, and look at what they gained in return. They became the king's right-hand men to help govern and rule the kingdom.

Every one of us has great potential to be successful in God and in life. God has endowed us with gifts and talents, and many times as believers, we fail to look at the word of God for success. Joshua 1:8 states: "This book of the law shall not depart out of thy mouth; but thou shalt meditate therein day and night, that thou mayest observe to do according to all that is written therein: for then thou shalt make thy way prosperous, and then thou shalt have good success." Daniel understood and believed in the promises of God to be successful.

We all have the freedom to choose what we want to do, how we are going to do it, and what we will and won't do. But I want to caution you about something: there is a price attached to the choice you make. From time to time I have had conversations with people who say that they don't have time for eating healthy because they are on the run and it's expensive. Well, it's better that you pay now, or else you'll pay later on the operating table, and it's just a matter of prioritizing your time to eat well.

I like to give a strategy that you can use because I stated earlier that it takes some personal effort and strategy to achieve your goal. On my job we have a store that we built up over time, and we sell candy bars, chips, soda, etc. To be honest with you, I like to eat some candy, chips, and soda, but I set a limit on that, especially at work. When work is slow, we tend to start eating things we have no business eating, and that's where we can get into big trouble. My strategy is to bring enough healthy snacks to eat throughout the workday to prevent me from eating the unhealthy junk food that I crave. I usually bring an apple, banana, nuts, grapes, yogurt, and trail mix bars of some kind, to just name a few. This type of eating keeps me in line with my diet and because I'm a runner certain foods that I eat helps me to perform well. If I eat the wrong things and go exercise, I feel it immediately, so I quickly learned to listen to my body about what I eat and how I feel. You can do this. Yes, I know it takes time and involves trial and error about what works and what doesn't work. God wants us to be disciplined and have control of our physical bodies for his glory.

Paul makes a very good statement about personal discipline and self control:

> Know ye not that they which run in a race run all, but one receives the prize? So run, that ye may obtain. And every man that strives for the mastery

is temperate in all things. Now they do it to obtain a corruptible crown; but we an incorruptible. I therefore so run, not as uncertainly; so fight I, not as one that beat the air: But I keep under my body, and bring it into subjection: lest that by any means, when I have preached to others, I myself should be a castaway. (1 Corinthians 9:24–27) KJV

Discipline is not always easy, in fact, it's sometimes uncomfortable and unpleasant, but the benefit in what it yields is what's important. When you keep yourself subjected to a healthy program, you become a product of that program, and you reap the benefits of that program.

I mentioned earlier about words like *wholesome, nourishing, fortified,* and *enrichment.* These descriptive words define the meaning of what is good for the body. These definitions are vital for us to understand the meaning of physical and spiritual nutrition for the body. When you read the definitions, you think about something natural, but while you are reading them, think what nourishes the soul so that it can be in good condition. This is bringing a new way of thinking spiritually how you feed your spirit, and it also changes your concepts of spiritual well-being.

These words support and give value to the meaning of *nutrition*:

- Wholesome—conducive to or suggestive of good health and physical well-being.
- Nourishment—the food or other substances necessary for growth, health, and good condition.
- Fortified—strengthened (a place) with defensive works so as to protect it against attack. Food fortification or enrichment is the process of adding micronutrients (essential trace elements and vitamins) to food.
- Enrichment—the process of adding nutrients to cereals or grain.

What's very important to remember is that eating a variety of good, nutritious foods is a preventive habit in that it keeps a lot of diseases and sickness under control. Some foods can fight off infections, and some can build your immune system over time. That doesn't mean that you won't get sick; it means that your body develops the ability to fight off infections, and you will be able to recover faster because you have fortified yourself with the essential vitamins and minerals.

Knowledge and understanding of food have been on the increase, which is causing people to be aware of their health and how food affects their bodies. Years ago I didn't worry about what I ate because I was so active in sports and growing up in my neighborhood. Being a typical adventurous young man, I could eat anything, and it never caused me to gain weight; nor did I have a serious health issue. I'm not that way now. I have to use wisdom and be very strategic to maintain my health and fitness as I get older. My eating habits play a major role in my being healthy and fit for many reasons, and it's a way of life for me.

Another issue I want to discuss is the issue of dieting—another misunderstood word when dealing with eating right. *Diet* (noun) means the kinds of food that a person, animal, or community habitually eats. For example, when you watch a nature show about the eating habits of bears, the narrator may say that the bear's *diet* consists of plants, berries, fish, and small mammals. I have put emphasis on the word habitually, because diet by definition means our way of eating, which is a big part of our lifestyle. The diet also means a special course of food to which one restricts oneself, either to lose weight or for medical reasons. This is very important because when an individual decides to make changes in their eating habits to be healthy, a controlled nutrition program is very important for that person to improve their health, and it is effective if they use it correctly.

Becoming educated in nutrition and understanding what's best for you is the best course of action to take when working to lose weight or for medical reasons. People have bought into many diet fads without any knowledge or guidance on developing good eating habits, and as a result of their ignorance they grow disappointed and discouraged. Sometimes people do more damage than good to their bodies because of the lack of knowledge and understanding.

What does the word of God say about lack of knowledge and understanding? "My people are destroyed from lack of knowledge" (Hosea 4:6 NIV). "Wisdom the principal thing; therefore get wisdom. And in all your getting, get understanding" (Proverbs 4:7 NKJV). We must depend on wisdom in every area of life. Wisdom only means the ability to apply knowledge, and that ability comes from faith in the word of God. Faith that acted upon will bring about the results you want because you are applying the word of God by his power. God is concerned about every fiber of our being so ask him to help, and listen, and then he will show you. Now that you have some information on dieting you don't have to cut back on eating; you just need to make better choices in your food. Develop a habit of understanding information and how it's good for you.

Being in good physical shape is a major demand in the military. One measure of its importance is a restructuring of the military to lay stress on members' physical condition, checking whether they are fit for duty. Soldiers are being evaluated for their level of fitness, and if they don't meet the standards, they are discharged from the military. The major health concern is being overweight, and its cause is eating unhealthy foods that lead to diminished health. We were told we would be either a liability or an asset based on our own choices if we wanted to stay in the military. This is serious, and this is someone's career.

Not only am I writing this through inspiration, but I am writing because I am concerned for the health of people's lives. Enjoy eating food, and on occasion have a cheat day and eat what you want. Just control yourself, be well-balanced in what you eat, and you will be all right. Evaluate yourself, and find out what's good for you and what's not. God wants us to be temperate in all things and he also wants us to enjoy the things he made—even *food*! Stay focused, and lean on God's ability to help. The scripture says: "I can do all things through Christ who strengthens me" (Philippians 4:13 NKJV).

One thing I've learned is that help comes from many sources. You have a heavenly Father you can commune with every day; you have people that God will lead you to who have experience and knowledge and can put you on the right path to your physical health. I will keep stressing that you can do this according to the word of God that you stand on. Please don't make excuses; we make time for many other things and fail to prioritize in our lives what is really important. Don't wait when until it's too late for you to realize that you have the power and the opportunity to do something about it right now!

I know that it gets hard sometimes to stay focused, and yes, I have to admit that Krispy Kreme, Oreo cookies, and the brownies à la mode get me every now and then. I love to eat! But I developed a disciplined philosophy about eating things like that; I call it the "do the crime, do the time" mentality, That means that if I eat such things, I have to hit the pavement, and I run five to ten miles, because my running schedule requires me to run long distance for endurance training, and I burn an estimated 500 to 1,000 calories for that workout. That's my strategy; in your case, you may have to avoid bad food altogether. It depends on your personal lifestyle. So although I'm being humorous, it's true that we all have our weaknesses, and really, that's okay as long as you can control those cravings and burn them efficiently.

What's wonderful is that when you do develop the disciplined lifestyle, you will have even more joy in eating these delicious treats, I certainly do without any guilt at all. As a matter of fact, I just ate a Twix candy bar while writing this book LOL!!! How about that? It's all in the knowledge and perspective when approaching the subject of health and how it can be beneficial to your life when you have the right information and the right concepts to apply it to your life.

You see how knowledge and wisdom can bring about a freedom in your life?

Once you experience this freedom, it's wonderful, and you almost feel guilty that you are eating these things and they don't affect you. Now you're surprised that you are not gaining weight because of your level of activity, and that is just awesome! Eat and eat well; be happy, and you will be a healthy, happy person. Have a balanced understanding about your perspective on life itself.

Eating is one of the main if not the main lifestyle habit in our lives. When we go on a vacation, we try to find entertainment and attractions, and most of the time they involve some type of reputable places to eat. We call ahead, or when we check into the hotel or resort, we ask the locals about the best places to eat, and most of the time the food is not healthy to eat, but it tastes so good! Right? Yes, I know I become a victim to the excitement of a vacation!

So have fun; eat, but don't put yourself under bondage especially when you are on vacation. When you are done, get back on track, and work hard to develop and maintain your eating habits. Believe me the benefits are very rewarding. When you go to the doctor and the numbers look very good or at least improved, you can feel good about yourself that you are doing something right. That becomes your motivation to maintain that healthy level of living.

3

JESUS, THE GREAT PHYSICIAN

The Spirit of the Lord is upon me, because he has
anointed me to preach the gospel to the poor; he
hath sent me to heal the brokenhearted, to preach
deliverance to the captives, and recovering of sight to
the blind, to set at liberty them that are bruised.

—Luke 4:18 (listing five spiritual conditions
due to the fall of mankind)

In the first couple of chapters we dealt with our physical health,
which we know is an important part of our lives. We need to
understand that we can't be so heavenly-minded that we are no
earthly good. Remember, our lives have to have balance, and even
when it comes to spiritual things, we can get to be so spiritual that
we rule out the physical dimension. But the spiritual dimension is
very important in understanding how we are to have a relationship
with Jesus Christ, and the only way is through his word.

Let's look at the greatest man that ever walked on this earth,
Jesus; no other human being that ever lived accomplished more
than he did, and rightfully so. He's is God in human flesh, and

God saw that it was necessary to come in a human form so we can understand who he is. He is the source of our spiritual health and strength, and as he said without him we can do nothing. Jesus is our Healer, Physician, and Strength. Everything we need is found in him and him only. Jesus came to heal and to save people's souls. He also came because he knew the condition of man in his sinful state (see Luke 4:18; 5:27–32).

Physicians know the condition of the human body and know how to heal it or treat the condition because they are educated, trained, qualified, and they have practiced their profession for years. Jesus knows the condition of human souls because he made them, and he knows every part of us. In fact, God qualified him and made him an all-sufficient Healer and Savior of the world (Luke 4:18). When he was on earth, he healed people physically so he could later heal them spiritually.

Jesus proclaimed to the Jewish community at that time that he was the anointed one prophesied by Isaiah, and he quoted Isaiah's prophecy concerning him. Part of that prophecy was that Jesus categorized the conditions of humankind, and with each condition he specifically stated what he would do about it. We take a careful approach in this passage of scripture to see how he is the source and power of our healing. Jesus never stated his own power that he was doing the work; he acknowledged that the Spirit of God was upon him and had anointed him for his earthly ministry. He knew the source of his power, and he even said (paraphrased), "The work that I do are not mine, but the Father in me he is doing the works."

We will take a look at Luke 4:18 to get a good understanding of each phrase. I want you to understand that each phrase is very significant, in that the Jesus is describing each spiritual and physical condition in nature. Although we may look okay on the outside, Jesus is able to look at the spiritual condition in all of us, and he shows us that he is the Great Physician of our souls and that we fell into one (or more) of these conditions. Let's explore the passage and explain what they mean:

The Spirit of the Lord is upon me, because he has anointed me

The first part of this passage of scripture states the "The Spirit of the Lord is upon me, because he has anointed me." The key word here is the anointing; without the anointing there is no effectiveness in your walk of life or your ministry. We sing a song that says the anointing makes the difference. There are people who go to church who don't have an anointed life. They are sweet people, but they don't operate in a way for the anointing to work in their life. The anointing has an amazing effect on how you live and how you do things.

What makes the anointing work is faith and prayer in the word of God. When you continue to feed your faith, you feed and energize the anointing in your life. Jesus made this declaration that the Spirit of God was on him and that God enabled him to do the work that he was about to announce. Notice that he said that the Spirit of the Lord was upon him first before announcing what his ministry would do. He recognized the anointing which gave the power and ability to take care of physical and spiritual conditions that have plagued humankind ever since the fall in the garden. Everything done in the believers' life must be done by his Spirit and faith activates and causes God to move for anything to be done.

Jesus was now proclaiming that this anointed power was about to be manifested in him. In the Old Testament there were times when the Spirit of God moved on a king, a prophet, or a servant of God, and through the power of God they did incredible exploits. God was about to do something extraordinary in the lives of people in the days that Jesus walked the earth, and it was about to be done through him. Jesus knew the Father was with him in everything that he was doing and that the results would bring deliverance to the people.

Jesus came to save the souls of men and women, and like a physician he knew that their condition was not only physical but spiritual as well. He saw the effects of sin that came into the world, and like a physician who is able to diagnose a bodily condition and treat it, Jesus is able to diagnose the condition of a soul and heal it with his anointed power. The scripture says that "God anointed Jesus of Nazareth with the Holy Ghost and with power: who went about doing good, and healing all that were oppressed of the devil; for God was with him" (Acts 10:38).

Jesus knew that he had a mission to complete before he knew that he had to die for the sins of the world. When he launched out in his ministry, it was a ministry of reconciliation and restoration. The Father have always been with him doing the dynamic ministry of healing people. What I have come to notice is that during Jesus' earthly ministries, he was showing us snapshots of what the kingdom of God will be like by healing people. From this example we can rest assured that in the kingdom every believer will be perfectly healthy and completely restored.

I just want to make very clear that it is Jesus who is the focus of our faith and the power comes from him. Everything was put into his hands to execute the will of the Father (God), and now through Jesus, he is the only one who is anointing all who believe in him to heal the sick. Look at the apostles in the book of Acts; they received this anointing power just as Jesus had, and they did what Jesus had done. To the point where is says in the scriptures that they turned the world upside down, there anointing had that effect on the people. Also, just as the Father was with Jesus, so Jesus was with the apostles: "And the hand of the Lord was with them: and a great number believed, and turned unto the Lord" (Acts 11:21), which means the anointing of the Lord was with them to do ministry and to carry out the mission of the Lord.

Believing has tremendous power. When you believe and operate in faith, the anointing will come to perform exploits like those of the apostles. As Jesus was anointed by the Father, so are we anointed by the Son.

Preach the gospel to the poor

God's concern for the poor is abundant in the pages of scripture because poverty results primarily from the unrighteous and the wicked conduct of either the poor individuals or the larger community. Poverty is also the result of oppression by people who can take advantage of people or a community who can't defend themselves because they lack the resources to do something about it.

To be *poor* is to lack sufficient money to live at a standard considered comfortable or normal in a society. Related words and phrases include *poverty-stricken, penniless, moneyless, impoverished, low-income, necessitous, impecunious, indigent, needy, destitute, pauperized,* and *unable to make ends meet.* When people are poor, they are subject to being constantly victimized due to their lack of resources; they basically are a help to nobody.

Why would anybody want to be around people with that condition? This mentality describes how most people look at the poor. Because if they are poor, then they live in poverty-stricken or very low-income housing, and this is not attractive to people who want to visit a city or a country. Those who counsel traveling safety often say: "Avoid poverty-stricken, low-income housing areas (projects/ghettos)." This poor environment breeds all kinds of domestic violence. Often people who come from such an environment are not educated, they look bad, and they are either angry or in much despair. I have been in some of these areas, and the people don't look happy.

Jesus told us to help feed the poor natural food and spiritual food as well. One passage of scripture tells a great story about helping somebody in need physically and spiritually, so Jesus knows of the balance of both. He knows that natural sustenance has been just as important as spiritual sustenance.

This is looking at the definition of *poor* from a physical sense; now let's look at it in a spiritual sense.

What type of poor is Jesus talking about? He is talking about being poor spiritually. "Blessed are the poor in spirit: for theirs is

35

the kingdom of heaven" (Matthew 5:3). Lacking the knowledge and understanding to apply the word of God will make you poor in the spirit. Your spirit lacks the spiritual sustenance from the word of God to be victorious in life. "Poor in the spirit" is a condition of the heart. We see people every day who let the world, beat them up because they don't have the spiritual fortitude to fight back against life's challenges.

Before I began to comprehend and understand these concepts of faith, I suffered spiritually in this area. I was poor in knowledge; in other words, I was ignorant of applying the word of God, and I suffered for it. Then I learned a whole new meaning of the word *gospel*. It means "good news," and most churches think that this is talking about what Jesus did on the cross. The gospel is any revelation revealed from God's word that you were not aware of— any insight made known to you as good news from the word that the Lord revealed to you to believe. When you act on this good news and let it change your thinking, then you have the knowledge to apply and use it to deliver you from the bondage of poverty. To be set free from this poor mentality, you must change your way of thinking, and the knowledge of the word of God is the only powerful way to make such changes.

Naturally, we have found ourselves in situations where we have suffered, in most cases due to fault of our own. Staying in a state of ignorance, which is a lack of knowledge and understanding, can harm us. When you have been in situations when you don't know what to do, your ignorance can lead to your own destruction. That's why the knowledge of the word of God needs to be taught—and you may notice that I didn't say *preached*. We must be taught and instructed in the word of God to show us that we can come out of a poor state of mind and tap into the blessings of God, who is able to make us rich in him.

When you are being taught and trained in faith concepts in the scriptures, you are not in the majority. A whole lot of church people are not being taught and instructed in the scriptures. They are what

I call spiritually sedentary; they just go to church, and they are churched, not taught.

The building block of the human soul is a daily diet of the word of God. We need to develop our spirits to be rich in faith to apply the truth and be delivered from a poor mindset. Knowledge will free us if we apply it to our lives. The scripture says, "Let the word of Christ dwell in you richly in all wisdom; teaching and admonishing one another in psalms and hymns and spiritual songs, singing with grace in your hearts to the Lord" (Colossians 3:16). When this scripture is made alive in your spirit, you have no lack because you are rich in faith. You now have the resources of faith in God's word to have whatsoever you say. You now have the capacity to speak to your poverty, and those faith-filled words will cause your situation to change. Begin to speak like God; God spoke things into existence by the power of his word. When you speak the word, you speak abundance into your life. There has to be an abundance in your spirit first, because when you are spiritually poor, you don't have the resources to draw upon. But when you have the abundance of faith-filled words in your spirit, then the power of activating those words will give you, the anointing (God's enablement) to free you from the poverty mindset. This is the teaching of Jesus that is delivering you from the bondage of poverty.

Heal the brokenhearted

Psalm 147:3 "He heals the brokenhearted and binds up their wounds" (Psalm 147:3 NKJV). "The LORD is near to the brokenhearted and saves the crushed in spirit" (Psalm 34:18 ESV). A broken heart (or heartbreak) is a common metaphor for the intense emotional pain or suffering one feels after losing a loved one, whether through death, divorce, breakup, physical separation, betrayal, or romantic rejection. Heartbreak is usually associated with losing a family member or spouse, though it can "break one's heart" to lose a parent, child, pet, a lover, or close friend, and it is frequently experienced during grief and bereavement. The phrase refers to the physical pain one may feel in the chest as a result of the loss, although by extension it includes the emotional trauma of loss even where it is not experienced as somatic pain. Although "heartbreak" ordinarily does not imply any physical defect in the heart, there is a condition known as "Takotsubo cardiomyopathy" (broken heart syndrome) in which a traumatizing incident triggers the brain to distribute chemicals that weaken heart tissue.

Heartbreak is a serious, deep hurt, and this type of hurt has led to suicides, murders, and many other tragic outcomes. When it happens, the negative result is anguish, the disappointment, or betrayal in the person's life. You also see the many family and friends who are greatly affected by such tragedies. It's difficult to try to help when you don't know how to help, unless you've been in that situation. What I have noticed is that when a person undergoes a heartbreak like divorce or the loss of someone, they try to do things to make up for that loss. Some try to take on a new hobby, they get very religious, or they become either very nice or very bitter, trying to vent and express what's inside.

What makes it so severe is when two lives that were joined together in holy matrimony and then for some reason are torn apart, they still take each other's life into another relationship. Even if they don't get into another relationship, they go their separate ways still influenced by each other, because they remain connected to each other, and God sees them as one flesh. When you rip flesh apart, it hurts. I can't imagine how a person must feel when the pain is so overwhelming that it seems God can't help, but please believe me when I tell you this: *"Yes, he can!"* With so much overwhelming grief and despair against you in situations like this, it seems that you can't win, and you feel defeated. Every one of us has been through some type of heartbreak in our lives, and we have felt the pain of it that can be overwhelming. I know I have.

When Jesus comes into your life the first thing he wants to do is heal your heart. Then he fills your heart with his words, and when they are faith-filled words, the heart is healed by faith in those words. This is an awesome work that you can't see with your eyes; it is a knowing in the spirit that true comfort has come to you. Naturally speaking, you can't tell whether an individual's heart is healthy or not. When you find out that something is wrong with your heart, you try to find out all the different ways to improve your heart health to prevent heart disease, a stroke, or a heart attack. So you improve your nutrition intake, you see a doctor, and you will notice a change in the way your body feels. What you are experiencing is a healing and relief of the heart because the right truths are being applied to your life. The same thing happens spiritually when you feed your heart the word of God—that is, the words of life and faith. Faith-filled words have to enter your heart, and when you fill your heart with the word of God, your faith activates the power of the word, which is the anointing that will bring the healing of the broken heart.

Remember to heed the sayings of Jesus written in the New Testament. As Charles Capps puts it, "All we have to do is read what is said in red and do what it says." Listen to what he says about letting the words affect your spirit: "It is the spirit that quickeneth; the flesh profiteth nothing: the words that I speak unto you, they are spirit, and they are life" (John 6:63). The scripture says that the life of all flesh is in the blood (see Leviticus 17:14). So it is with the word of God: the life of the Spirit of God is in the word because the word is living and powerful (see Hebrews 4:12).

This is one thing that I know: when the word is believed by faith it works. I remember going through some heartbreaks, and I've found that when I was faced with dealing with the situations on my own, I recalled the promises of God's word for my situation and for my life. This is the secret to being successful in being healed from heartbreak: "Put the word of God in your heart."

Preach deliverance to the captives

Deliverance is the action of being rescued or set free through "prayers for deliverance." There are other words that are similar in meaning to clarify the word *deliverance*: liberation, release, delivery, discharge, rescue, emancipation; salvation. It may be a formal or authoritative utterance used to proclaim or announce something. Let's explain this issue of deliverance, which even after salvation, there are some things in our lives that we must be delivered from. So don't fool yourself by thinking that even after salvation, everything is all right, and you are whole. I'm not trying to be the bearer of bad news, but it is a fact of life.

Yes, it is true that a finished work was completed on the cross by Jesus—a spiritual work to bring salvation to the world. But the process is that we must make that a reality in our lives by putting our trust in what was done on the cross; as the scriptures say, "Leaving the principles of the doctrine…, let us go on unto perfection" (Hebrews 6:1). So we know about the finished work on the cross; we need to believe the rest of the word of God dealing with issues in our lives that can still keep us in bondage and ignorance.

I remember talking with my father-in-law about this issue of deliverance, and he told me that there are people who come to church and put on a front as if everything is all right, rather than coming to the reality that they need to be delivered from some things. We can be right here in church fooling ourselves that we don't need deliverance from some bad habits we develop in life. Yes, we have salvation, but we need deliverance to. If we don't need deliverance from bad habits and bad thinking, why did God not let the Bible stop at the gospels? Why the epistles? Why are there letters to the church? We still need to be refined and gain the victory over personal battles in our lives. Christ has to present us faultless to the Father. Did he not say that we are over comers by the word of our testimony and by the blood of the lamb? So we have to be delivered from some things. Another reason is that we can become useful for the Lord's use in ministering the word of God to people that are hurting and held captive by their problems. The gospels are like the Declaration of Independence: they give the teaching and preaching of our Lord Jesus, which are the foundation of the Christian life. The epistles (letters) give the laws for righteous living.

Captives are people who are held in bondage or imprisonment. The word describes one held in the grip of a strong emotion or passion based on what is in their mind and heart. One doesn't have to be in a prison or jail to be captive or held in bondage. We can be held in bondage to our own thinking. Even in the comforts of our own home, we can be held captive or in bondage to habits we've developed in our lives. For example, food is a slave master to some people, and it's their bondage.

When people walk in ignorance, they are in bondage because they are unable to come out of what they are in. Do you know that ignorance is a type of bondage? When you don't know anything, you are stuck, and can't get out, and you are held captive by your own ignorance. I have been told that some of the people I grew up with are not doing so well in life because of their mentality. One day I had a thought, looking at some of the people I knew, and I realized, *They are stuck, and they can't get out or move up in life.*

I call it being environmentally institutionalized. This sounds like a big, educated phrase, but it's very simple. Being institutionalized is the psychological and mental health effect of living for a long time in an institution or similar facility. *Environmentally institutionalized* is a mind-set that affects people in a community who can't seem to move up in life. Either they are comfortable where they are, or they fear to move from their surroundings. The problem is that they are oppressed by being uneducated; to put it in simple terms, they are ignorant, with no exposure to learning things to improve their lives. This type of syndrome we see in the people we love. There are people who love to stay around the familiar all their lives and never want to explore and see the wonderful things that God has provided for their lives. They are held captive, by their own choice.

God has provided a way out of that captive mind-set through knowledge of the glorious gospel of Jesus Christ. When we hear the gospel and respond to it by faith, an amazing process begins to take place in our hearts. Jesus said he would "preach deliverance to the captives." How is that done? There are people who grew up in a poverty-stricken neighborhood who at a young age have been inspired to learn, and that learning was their ticket out of poverty because the knowledge they acquired made that happen for them. So if a student who lives in such an environment is very good at mathematics, for example, a teacher may see that gift and inspire the student to excel in that area. Once students catch on to the possibilities out there, then they can achieve the impossible because of knowledge—and not just knowledge alone but the application of that knowledge. It's that individual's ticket out of a bad environment.

Similarly, when we hear the gospel of Jesus Christ, obtain knowledge of the word of God, and act on it by faith, then we can be delivered from bad habits of sin that holds us captive. Because faith in the word of God activates a power in us to be delivered, what we will begin to experience is the law of faith. The law of faith supersedes the law of sin. When we operate by the law of faith, we are lifted above that captivity and bondage, and we are set free. It is the law of faith that frees us from that captive, slave mentality mind-set. When you experience the awesome power of God delivering you, it is absolutely amazing, just because you believe what was preached. It's not just preached; it's preached with power to save and deliver.

It is faith together with knowledge of the truth that makes you free. "Then said Jesus to those Jews which believed on him, If ye continue in my word, then are ye my disciples indeed; and ye shall know the truth, and the truth shall make you free" (John 8:31–32). This passage of scripture is showing us that there are conditions for deliverance and freedom. The Lord said that truth will make you free, so we need to see that the truth of the word of God has creative ability to give us freedom. This truth has got to be birthed in your spirit; in other words, it has become a reality in your spirit that you are free. I hope you are seeing the message because God is pouring this message into your spirit to feed your faith with the knowledge of his will to save you, deliver you, and make you whole for his glory and purpose. This is Jesus doing the work, so always remember who your deliverer is. Jesus is the only one that can bring freedom to your soul when it's damaged and in bondage to sin.

Recovering of sight to the blind

Recovering is a return to a normal state of health, mind, or strength. Blindness is the condition of lacking visual perception due to physiological or neurological factors. Various scales have been developed to describe the extent of vision loss and define blindness. Total blindness is the complete lack of form and visual light perception and is clinically recorded as NLP, an abbreviation for "no light perception." Blindness is frequently used to describe severe visual impairment with residual vision. Those described as having only light perception have no more sight than the ability to tell light from dark and the general direction of a light source.

According to this scripture, it's the restoring of one's sense of perception that has been darkened by sin. It's a dulled spiritual perception. A person who can't see is seeing nothing but darkness, having no ability to see anything or perceive anything. The story in Mark 10:46–52 of Jesus healing Bartimaeus brings out a great illustration and an analogy about the subject of restoring a blind man's sight. Bartimaeus knew that he needed help, and he heard about Jesus coming by where he was and cried out to Jesus for help. The commotion got Jesus' attention, so that he stood still and called to the blind man. Jesus told the man before he healed him to go his way; his faith had made him whole.

What is the key to this passage of scripture? Bartimaeus heard and believed, and when he called out to Jesus, he knew that he would be healed. Why? Jesus was attracted to the faith of Bartimaeus; that's why he stood still and called to the man, because the man called on the Lord for healing. What does the scripture say? "Faith comes by hearing, and hearing by the word of God" (Romans 10:17 NKJV). Now Bartimaeus received healing for a physical ailment, but used a spiritual principle to get results in the natural.

My wife and I were discussing this topic found in 2 Corinthians 4 concerning the condition of people who are blind spiritually and what we found was very enlightening. The scripture says, "But if our gospel be hid, it is hid to them that are lost: In whom the god of this world hath blinded the minds of them which believe not, lest the light of the glorious gospel of Christ, who is the image of God, should shine unto them" (2 Corinthians 4:3–4). I want to call your attention to the phrase in this passage, "blinded the minds"; this very passage jumps off the page and into our hearts about how a person's mind is blinded. This is very disturbing: when you are blind and you don't know it, you are in a world of trouble, having lost your perception and your ability to discern. You are walking in darkness, which really means you are walking in ignorance. The devil's job as the prince of darkness is to keep us in ignorance and, if he can, to keep us from knowing the truth. Then we become his victims so he can destroy us. What's the saying? "What you don't know will kill you or hurt you."

But there is good news in the rest of this passage of scripture, and that is the "light of the glorious gospel of Christ." That light is the revelation of the knowledge of Jesus Christ; when it is received in your spirit, that is the recovering of sight to the blind mind. Knowledge of the word eliminates the darkness, which means you have knowledge, and ignorance is done away with. When you go into a dark room and turn on the light, what happens to the darkness? The light also makes you aware of what's in the room. If there is a something dangerous in the room, such as a hole in the floor, and the lights are out, you are not aware of the hazard that can harm you. But when there is light, you are aware of the hazards and the pitfalls that are there. Light makes us aware of how much we need a savior and a deliverer.

Second Corinthians 6:14 (AMP) read, "Do not be unequally yoked with unbelievers [do not make alliances with them or come under a different yoke with them, inconsistent with your faith]. For what partnership have right living and right standing with God with iniquity and lawlessness? Or how can light have fellowship with darkness?" What does the scripture say? Light and darkness can't cohabit together; one has got to go, so make sure it's the darkness. Revelation knowledge illuminates our spirit, and we are made aware of our sinfulness. Then we can cry out to the Lord like Bartimaeus, knowing that we need healing to recover our sight.

Jesus is the light of the world; he is the one who reveals to us who we really are through knowledge of his word. We must have a born-again experience to have the capacity to contain the knowledge of God. Jesus said that you must be born again to even see the kingdom, so without the spiritual new birth, you will be in darkness. If you can't see, then your perception of spiritual things is clouded with human reasoning and philosophy. There has to be a regeneration of the mind and heart to see and experience the life in the knowledge of the word of God. Jesus is the only one that can recover our spiritual sight to focus on him. Scripture says, "This is the message we have heard from him and proclaim to you, that God is light, and in him is no darkness at all. If we say we have fellowship with him while we walk in darkness, we lie and do not practice the truth. But if we walk in the light [revelation knowledge] as he is in the light, we have fellowship with one another, and the blood of Jesus his Son cleanses us from all sin" (1 John 1:5–7 ESV).

To set at liberty them that are bruised

This phrase means to put a person in a state of freedom from injury. Liberty is the state being free within society from oppressive restrictions imposed by authority on one's way of life, behavior, or political views. Bruised means having suffered an injury that is causing discoloration of the skin; the outward appearance reflects the damage that is internal. This also tells us that we don't know how severe the damage is; the reason for the discoloration is the crushed blood vessels underneath the skin.

I like to bring out a natural illustration about scripture for us to see the spiritual implication of this text. Jesus said "set at liberty," which means to place in a position to be free from injury or harm. This shows us that he will specifically put us in a place where we have freedom to worship and commune with him and be healed internally in our spirit.

Several scriptures come to mind when I think about this text. Second Corinthians 3:17 (NIV) states, "Now the Lord is the Spirit, and where the Spirit of the Lord is, there is freedom [liberty]." An amazing thing happens when there is a spiritual rebirth or born-again experience that happens after salvation of the soul, namely that God puts us in Christ. Jesus literally baptizes us and puts us in his body, and there is liberty (freedom) in the body of Christ. Jesus is specific when saying "set at liberty," which means that by his grace he has positioned us in a place in him to be free. This work of Christ is something that causes you to be free, and it's done by his Spirit through faith in him and him alone.

Second Corinthians 5:17 states, "Therefore if any man be in Christ, he is a new creature: old things are passed away; behold all things are become new." I want to bring out another issue concerning this freedom, and that is we are free from the man-made traditions and religious legalism. Jesus always had conflict with the religious authorities during his time on earth. If there is a condition in the church that is worse than any other, it is being spiritually bruised by leadership doctrine, and sometimes it is self-inflicted. There are people in churches who have been brutally hurt by toxic leadership, and their true situation is that they are in bondage and can't enjoy living for God because of the power of legalistic doctrine. Sometimes the hurt is so damaging that it's unspeakably what leaders have done to church members. Doctrine is powerful, and it has the ability to put people in bondage.

God has called us to freedom, but for some reason man has failed to teach God's people that we are free and have only one master. We have added our own philosophy to the scriptures, and we have tainted the word of God to fit the way we want to interpret it. For example, one reason I like our church is the fact that we can dress casually or dress up, as long as it's decent, and with God's Spirit in us, we know better how to dress and not offend our brothers and sisters in Christ. Some churches are so traditional, they don't promote being romantic in marriage. This is very sad; this and other teachings have destroyed marriages and made them dull. If you have the Spirit of God in you, you know how to do right. Liberty doesn't mean that we have the freedom to do whatever we want; we are governed by the word of God, and his commandments cause us to behave in a manner that is pleasing to him. Yes, we have freedom, but we are ruled by the grace of God, not by intimidation.

Scripture says, "For God has not given us a spirit of fear, but of power and of love and of a sound mind" (2 Timothy 1:7 NKJV). When Jesus healed people, there was a release from whatever it was that had them in bondage, whether it was pain, sickness, or disease. God is a God who wants his children healed and made whole by the power of Jesus Christ through faith.

To end on this subject, I want you to always remember that the greatest healing that Christ can do for you is to heal you from the bondage of sin and all the damage that comes with sin. There is no sin so dreadful that he can't forgive it; there is no disease so severe that he can't heal it. Jesus died a dreadful death to bring salvation and healing to mankind and to deliver us from the curse of sin. Just like the physician who wants to bring healing and restore your health, Christ wants to restore your soul as well as your physical body, and he takes pleasure in doing this for all who put their faith in his teachings and his power.

Jesus Christ said, "The thief cometh not, but for to steal, and to kill, and to destroy: I am come that they might have life, and that they might have it more abundantly" (John 10:10). Jesus came that we might have abundant life now and later on for all eternity. God did not create human beings to be miserable. God created us to have a wonderful relationship with him and to enjoy the things he created for us to be happy.

4

THE CONDITION OF THE HEART

A good man out of the good treasure of his heart brings forth
good; and an evil man out of the evil treasure of his heart brings
forth evil. For out of the abundance of the heart his mouth speaks.

—Luke 6:45 (NKJV)

Keep your heart with all diligence, for out
of it spring the issues of life.

—Proverbs 4:23 (NKJV)

Do not be anxious about anything, but in every situation, by
prayer and petition, with thanksgiving, present your requests to
God. And the peace of God, which transcends all understanding,
will guard your hearts and your minds in Christ Jesus.

—Philippians 4:6–7 (NIV)

What's in your heart? Do you know that one of the most difficult
and humbling things for us to do is express what's in our hearts and
minds? After examining the two topics about the heart and mind,
I have to carefully explain what they are spiritually, because this

is the playing field where doctrine will reside and take root in our spirit. I had to break this up into two chapters to discuss in detail the condition of the heart and mind because this is where the battle is fought. We know that it starts in the mind and hearts of believers, and this is where God wants to deal with us when we come to him.

What does the scripture say in regard to what God sees in man?

> But the LORD said to Samuel, "Do not look at his appearance or at his physical stature, because I have refused him. For the LORD does not see as man sees; for man looks at the outward appearance, but the LORD looks at the heart." (1 Samuel 16:7 NKJV)

In spite of all the positions and prestigious influences of man's achievements, God still focuses on the heart. Listen up, people in leadership; he is not impressed with your position if your heart is not fixed on him. What did Jesus say? "Jesus said to him, 'You shall love the LORD your God with all your heart, with all your soul, and with all your mind'" (Matthew 22:37 NKJV).

The Heart

What's in your heart? We would all feel very uncomfortable to be put in the spotlight to express what's going on inside of us. Some would be surprised, embarrassed, ashamed, interesting, and sometimes humorous. Why? Because we would think people will think differently about us if we express what we really are and how it will affect the people we influence. Some people are free enough to express how they feel and even tell about the pitfalls and mistakes that they've made in life. When people speak, they are expressing what's in their hearts; as the Bible says, "Out of the abundance of the heart the mouth speaks" (see Matthew 12:34). It's a true statement, and given enough time to talk, people will eventually tell on themselves, and they will reveal what's in their heart when they get comfortable in the right environment.

This is why I want to deal with this heart and mind issue and how it affects our daily lives. Everybody on the face of this earth has a developed a mind-set, a heart for the things that are healthy or unhealthy, whether spiritual or physical. Our physical heart is the most essential organ in the body because it pumps blood to all the vital organs in the body. If the heart malfunctions, you are in trouble, and you are subject to heart conditions that can be fatal. Taking care of that ticker in their chest is the priority in a person's life once they find out that there is a problem in their condition that needs careful attention. We need to do the same with our spiritual heart and to see if we have a heart problem.

Just to add a note, doctors say that only thirty minutes a day of simply walking can prevent heart issues. Most of the time we are the major cause of our condition because we abuse our own bodies without a care in the world until they have us on an operating table with our chest cut open. Examine yourself, pause for a moment, and think... *Hmmm. Is this my fault? Did I bring this on myself physically and spiritually? Am I being deceived in the heart?* Don't look at anybody else, and don't think these words are for others; no, I'm talking about you! When we take a look at our health issues spiritually and physically, we realize that we have some fault. I remember the story of a man who was going to sue McDonald's for making him fat. Really? Nobody made him stuff his face with that junk food in the first place. Hello! Choices! We all have choices!

We bring these things on ourselves, thinking that there are no consequences for the choices we make, but there are. What made me think of this topic is that I went into a grocery store one day and picked up some health supplements and read some of the labels. They said they were for "heart health." The question in my mind was how they help the heart. Being a researching word nerd, I looked up the benefits of these supplements and found they offer tremendous benefits to the heart, blood, and circulatory system.

I had some health issues that needed some attention. To be honest with you, I'm not exempt either. I don't want you to think that I've graduated from health struggles; I have to practice what I preach too. Recall the testimony I gave at the beginning of this book of how I did something about my health. It wasn't serious, but it was enough of a wake up call for me to do something about it. I am always researching and finding out a better way of doing something. That's why my life is good: I've learned from people who know things. I'm still learning, and what's beneficial is not just to learn, but to apply the learning. Now I'm talking about the physical part of heart health, but I want you to see the physical so you can see and understand this analogy spiritually.

Before I purchased those supplements, I educated myself on what I was putting in my body and the benefits the supplements offered. We know that by definition the heart is a muscle in the chest that pumps blood, nutrients, and oxygen to all parts of the body for normal, healthy bodily functions. Spiritually speaking, the heart is really who you are, and we can observe that how people act is the result of what's in their heart. When a person's conversation is filthy, then their heart is filthy, and their mind is darkened as well. Scripture teaches that "out of the heart are the issues of life" (see Proverbs 4:23), and that's why we express our issues, whether good or bad. This is a good example; a person can improve their heart health by following simple guidelines from many different health sources. The point that I want you to see is that there are two sides to this improvement that are spiritual and natural. The same way I am showing that there are guidelines for natural improvement, there are guidelines and steps for the spiritual as well.

Let's take a look at the natural, and while we consider it, start thinking about examples of the spiritual that you are already familiar with in light of scripture to give you an understanding how we are to promote our practice of spiritual health. One website (http://health. clevelandclinic.org) lists seven steps you can take to improve heart health, and these are just the simple ways. These steps have a spiritual content to them if we pay attention to each step; that is, there is a scripture that supports each step and brings clarity to it: (1) Get active, (2) Control cholesterol, (3) Eat better, (4) Manage blood pressure, (5) Lose weight, (6) Reduce blood sugar, and (7) Stop smoking! Is this simple enough? Each step carries easy-to-explain benefits. If you want to improve your heart, this is what you do physically.

Now let's switch gears here. How do you improve your heart spiritually? We must see this in detail, and rightfully so, because of the important applications involved in developing a healthy spiritual life. Let's begin with this thought: "Everywhere we look today, we are bombarded with messages warning us of the importance of heart-healthy choices. What about the health of our spiritual heart? Would a spiritual cardiologist has reason to be concerned about the condition of your spiritual health?" I responded to that question by saying it depends on who is the spiritual cardiologist. I would make sure that my spiritual cardiologist is the Lord Jesus because nobody else qualifies for that position. Jesus states in scripture that he knows what's in a person's heart, and he knows the condition of the heart as nobody else does because he made it.

I'm going to list some steps or guidelines that can improve your spiritual heart, but are also valuable in showing you what you should avoid to protect your heart. Your heart is vital; it's the source of who you really are, but it is gullible and can be deceived if you let it. You are the defender of your heart, and this is the only time that you have a license to be righteously selfish about your heart. You have the right to choose healthiest things to eat, and sometimes, just as it can be annoying to hear people hound and tease you about what you eat, so it is with your spiritual heart. Don't let people pressure you into what they want you to hear; this is your soul, and you have the God-given right to decide how you want your heart developed into the word of God.

When we are sitting in churches week after week hearing biblical truths, are we letting God write them in our heart? I often wonder at the many attending church each Sunday, and I wonder to myself what type of heart that word is falling on. How the word of God affects your heart will determine how much you submit to it. Don't expose your heart to people; expose your heart to the revelation of scripture. Jesus said that his words are spirit and life to those who find them (see John 6:63). Letting God deal with our hearts and minds is a work of a lifetime while we are still on this earth. Nobody graduates from the constant work of Christ on your spirit. It's a consistent life of walking by faith in the word, but it has to be in your heart. You have to put this word in you. Your heart has to be ready to receive wholesome truth from the word of God. Just like the best natural supplements to benefit the natural heart, good supplements from the word of God will heal your heart.

The word of God is like a powerful cleansing agent in the heart. For example, garlic is a powerful herb. It is best known as a flavoring and seasoning for food. But over the years, garlic has been used as a medicine to prevent or treat a wide range of diseases and conditions. One of its benefits is that it helps to purify the blood, builds the immune system to fight off infections, and lowers blood pressure, helping to prevent heart disease. But you have to put this herb in you through food or take it as a dietary supplement to see the benefits. My point is that you have to put the word of God in you and let it purify your heart, and just as it can happen with our natural heart, sin has polluted and darkened our spiritual hearts. Just as it takes time to improve your heart health, it takes time to improve your spiritual health as well.

It's imperative that you take in the word of God through hearing, reading, and speaking these truths into your spirit. The scripture says, "Wherefore lay apart all filthiness and superfluity of naughtiness, and receive with meekness the engrafted word, which is able to save your souls" (James 1:21). Notice in this passage that there are conditions that you must follow if you want your heart cleansed by the word of God; it says to "lay aside all filthiness and sinful naughtiness" because this gets in the way. Why? Because it's a spiritual resistance to the knowledge of God, and God will not allow his word to be mixed with filth. The other part of this passage that brings light to our subject is the word *engrafted*, which means to firmly fix or engrave deeply into something. That's the attitude we must have when we receive the word of God in our spirit. Don't fool yourself thinking that you don't need heart help; we all do, some more than others. So our hearts need to be carefully examined by the word of God daily.

In Matthew 13:1–23, Jesus is teaching a parable of the sower (farmer), and he describes what happens when we hear the word of God, depending on what type of heart is receiving it. He describes four different heart types, which relate to all people. This illustration is how the seed of the word of God is planted into a person's heart and how each heart is affected by how they receive it. The passage speaks of four different types of people who Jesus is described as having one of these heart types that hears the word of the kingdom: I want you to see how the word of God represents seed, and how that seed is planted is what's important in this text. Always take into account how you hear the word of God.

In truth, you fall into one of these categories concerning how you are hearing, and this has an effect on your spiritual walk. Most of time our failure is that we are not hearing, and Jesus told us to let these sayings sink into our ears (Luke 9:44). Let's read the parable:

Parable of the Sower

> Behold, a sower [farmer] went out to sow, and as he sowed, some seed fell by the wayside; and the birds came and devoured them. Some fell on stony places, where they did not have much earth; and they immediately sprang up because they had no depth of earth. But when the sun was up they were scorched, and because they had no root they withered away. And some fell among thorns, and

the thorns sprang up and choked them. But others fell on good ground and yielded a crop: some a hundredfold, some sixty, some thirty. He who has ears to hear, let him hear! (Matthew 13:3–9 NKJV)

The Lesson about the Sower

Therefore hear the parable of the sower: When anyone hears the word of the kingdom, and does not understand it, then the wicked one comes and snatches away what was sown in his heart. This is he who received seed by the wayside. But he who received the seed on stony places, this is he who hears the word and immediately receives it with joy; yet he has no root in himself, but endures only for a while. For when tribulation or persecution arises because of the word, immediately he stumbles. Now he who received seed among the thorns is he, who hears the word, and the cares of this world and the deceitfulness of riches choke the word, and he becomes unfruitful. But he who received seed on the good ground is he who hears the word and understands it, which indeed bears fruit and produces: some a hundredfold, some sixty, some thirty. (Matthew 13:18–23 NKJV)

The Bible speaks a lot about the heart, and it describes many different types of hearts. The heart is the center of life itself, and when the heart dies, so does the body. Jesus describes how the word of God fell on four different types of hearts, and they all had one thing in common: they heard the word of the kingdom. But how was it received? Let's look at the types of hearts he describes:

❖ Fell by the wayside – This individual does not understand it, and the enemy takes it away from his heart. Note: The enemy's job is to take words from your heart!

❖ Fell into stony places – This person hears it with emotion and enjoys what he is hearing, but because his heart is not fertile enough to contain the word, he is always offended, and when troubles come, he fails, because the word of God is not rooted in him.

❖ Fell among thorns – This person receives the word, but his heart is toward the cares of worldly riches and wealth, which choke the word. The word can't work on him to produce fruit (godly character) because his heart is after worldly things and not after God.

❖ Fell into good ground – This person's heart has been broken by humility and submission to the word of God. His heart is very humble, and God is able to plant the seed of his word in his heart. As a result, he is blessed abundantly and producing the godly, righteous character as a result of receiving the word of God by faith.

The lesson of this parable is that each of us falls into one of these four groups. Which one are you? If you want your heart to be blessed by the word of God, make sure that your heart is good ground. Humble your heart so it can receive faith-filled words from the word of God. I have listed some guidelines to help us establish a healthy spiritual life that is pleasing to the Lord. Your spirit will be greatly blessed if you follow these basic guidelines.

Spiritual Guidelines for a Healthy Heart

❖ **Study the Word of God (Hebrews 2:15; James 1:21).** This is the number-one essential part of our spiritual development. It is by far the hallmark of our believing in what we put our faith in, and without it we fail. Why?

Because the scriptures say that "every word of God is pure" (Proverbs 30:5). It's full of faith and power. If you cut off the word supply, you will come down, just as an airplane comes down if you cut off its fuel supply. Strength comes from faith in the word (Hebrews 4:12). Confidence comes from faith in the word (Philippians 1:6). All our promises come from faith in the word (1 Corinthians 1:20). My mother shared with me a wonderful statement about the word of God: "If you feed your faith the word of God, you will starve your doubts to death." We have to study and meditate to put the word in us. What does the scripture say? "I seek you with all my heart; do not let me stray from your commands. I have hidden your word in my heart that I might not sin against you" (Psalm 119:10–11 NIV).

❖ **Hear the Word (Romans 10:17; Joshua 1:8).** This is just as essential as studying in the sense that you have to rehearse or play back in your mind what you've read and what you heard. Speak the word of God to yourself. Give voice to God's word. Make it a conscious effort to speak a word to your spirit. Find and listen to an excellent, faith-filled pastor whose teaching the word of God, and research and find good Bible teachers online, and read some of their literature. There are a lot of good ones out there, as well as a lot of bad ones. Thank God for the technology of recording tapes and CDs. When you meditate on the word of God, you are hearing it spiritually in mind and your heart receives. Always be ready to hear the word of God, and hear it with joy.

❖ **Have a Consistent Prayer Life (Philippians 4:6; Ephesians 6:18).** "Praying always with all prayer and supplication in the Spirit, and watching thereunto with all perseverance and supplication for all saints" (Ephesians 6:18). God wants us to have a prayer life, and it's essential to developing a relationship with him. He wants us to commune with him. We are talking to our heavenly Father. Prayer brings strength, and you can pray in many different ways, and he understands it all. Prayer guides you and give you a clear answer from the word of God. Prayer is the heartbeat of the anointing of God. Prayer gives you clear direction and understanding about how to handle a situation. Prayer quiets your spirit and brings peace in the midst of trouble. Prayer keeps us focused on the Lord Jesus because as the high priest, he prays and intercedes on our behalf to the Father (Hebrews 7:24–25; Romans 8:26).

❖ **Develop Your Faith (Hebrews 11:6).** The only way we can please God is by faith. Faith is the only thing that moves God. Jesus says, "Have faith in God" (Mark 11:22). You want God to be attracted to you, so move by faith and watch the dynamics of faith be performed in your life. Read the fourth chapter (Hebrews 11), and see how God blessed everyone that had faith in him. Christ was always moved by faith, and although he is dwelling in another dimension where we can't see him, he is still moved by faith. The Bible says that not all people have faith. That means that if they are not hearing the word of God and they don't have the knowledge of the word of God in them, then they don't have faith. Faith comes from hearing God's word, and if you do not hear God's word, faith is not coming (Romans 10:17). Here is the spiritual challenge, how do you live? By faith? Well, it better is based on information from the Word of God. Faith filled words has to enter your heart to see the dynamic power of God working in your life. Filling your heart with faith drives away fear and worry. That's why faith in the word of God must become a working knowledge of faith which is how faith is developed into the heart of the believer.

❖ **Develop Relationships with People of Faith.** This is one of the most important steps for every new believer coming into the body of Christ. My greatest blessing in growing in the word of God was being under the care of Spirit-filled, faith-filled, and Bible-knowledgeable mentors. You noticed how I described those mentors. Why? Scripture says this "Where no counsel is, the people fall: but in the multitude of counselors there is safety" (Proverbs 11:14). You need to develop a relationship with one or more people who know what they are talking about and have exercised themselves in the doctrine of the word of God. They become your spiritual guide(s) to keep you in line with scripture. Pay close attention to the passages of scripture concerning the type of people you need to be engaged in (for example, Hebrews 5:12–14). There are carnally minded people in church who operate in the flesh, and they are filled with garbage that you have to avoid. We're still dealing with the heart, so you have to guard your heart against fleshly minded people. These are toxic influences that you need to be aware of. When you begin to educate your spirit in the word of God, through prayer, God will enhance your discernment and awareness of these types of influences.

❖ **Avoid Carnally Minded People (Romans 8:6).** There is nothing worse for your spiritual health than fleshly, carnally minded so-called Christians. They walk after the dictates of their fleshly mind. They don't live like Christ! They don't benefit your spirit when it comes to spiritual matters. That's why the scripture says to "guard your heart with all diligence, for out of it are the issues of life" (Proverbs 4:23, paraphrased), because these types of people have ungodly issues and problems in which you don't want to be entangled. Be careful whom you spend time with because you don't know what people are involved with. I know from experience that some people are nothing but little devils used to infiltrate the body of Christ to spread their toxic agenda and fill your spirit with ungodly mess. Watch them carefully!

❖ **Know Your Enemy.** "Lest Satan should get an advantage of us: for we are not ignorant of his devices" (2 Corinthians 2:11). In the military, we are taught and trained to know the enemy by their size, capabilities, and location. Based on the information gathered by intelligence. We can mount an attack with the appropriate firepower, and in most cases we do so with an overwhelming force. The important thing is that you know your enemy, because your strongest weapon in fighting the enemy is knowledge. The enemy's job is to infiltrate into the minds and hearts of God's people. But the battle has to be fought with strategy. The word of God commands us to put on the whole armor of God, that we may be able to fight the enemy (see Ephesians 6:11). We as saints need to become spiritually intelligent in the word of God because there is a blessing in doing so. When our hearts are filled with the knowledge of God's word, then by faith we can guard our hearts with all diligence, we can hide the word in our hearts that we don't sin against our Lord, and our hearts will not be troubled because the peace of God will rule and keep our hearts right.

❖ **Beware of False Doctrine (Matthew 7:15–20).** An absolutely dangerous doctrine is being promoted in churches, and most churches are not aware of it. False teaching has plagued our churches for many years—in fact, from the beginning. Paul warned us to beware of the false teachers that would come in and lead people away from the truth. Be careful what you fill your heart with, because there is a great deception rooted in the false teaching, and many will be hurt and destroyed if they are not spiritually aware of it. The truth of biblical doctrine is the only way that we can know that false doctrine is being taught.

The scriptures, specifically tell us to study to show ourselves approved unto God, rightly dividing the word of truth (see 2

Timothy 2:15). When we exercise and develop our faith in the word of God, we can discern the enemy when he comes, and we can put up a defense against his devices and schemes.

What I wanted to bring out in this chapter is keys to protecting your heart and feeding your heart the right things that will promote a healthy spiritual life. Just as you eat healthy foods to take care of your heart, you also need spiritual food to take care of your spiritual heart. God wants to reside in our hearts, writing his wholesome words of faith there. When your heart is filled with his word, by faith, you will live out what is in your heart. The scripture says, "As a man thinks in his heart, so is he" (Proverbs 23:7, paraphrased). Remember the saying, "You are what you eat"; the same statement applies to our hearts: "you are what you think in your heart." It is up to us. God has given us a choice to serve him.

He knows the heart, and he is the only one who can calm a troubled heart by his peace. Christ is the only one who can see our hearts, and he knows the intentions of the heart. If there are things in your heart that you know are unrighteous, take them to the Lord. Yes, we can confess our faults to one another, but it is God who restores all hearts because the scriptures say that he is greater than our hearts, and we know that his grace is the only thing that is sufficient for our lives.

We considered the previous chapters how to make our natural hearts healthy, but do we know how to heal a spiritual heart? That's the question. It is not easy to do because you don't know what type of heart you are dealing with when it comes to people. People are finicky, and when you start dealing with someone's heart, it can be a sensitive, touchy subject. When dealing with different issues that affect us, like for example, racism, you begin to see what's inside of people when that topic comes up. You see the real person emerge. Controversy and conflict will bring out either the best or the worst in all of us. Most of the time it sits there dormant until certain buttons are pushed or we are put in certain situations. Pressure always reveals who we really are, and since most of us stay in our comfort zone, we prefer to be around the people we love, who have no issue with us.

One thing I've learned about this heart issue is that you can know where someone's heart is. Colossians 3:2 says, "Set your affection on things above, not on things on the earth." Affection is a gentle feeling of fondness or liking toward someone or something. Jesus states it this way: "For where your treasure is, there will your heart be also" (Matthew 6:21). What we treasure the most, such as our family, money and the things we possess, is what causes us to act a certain way because it represents what we are. Is Jesus sitting on the throne of your heart? Is he treasured more than anything else? When put in the right situations, this scripture challenges all of us to see whether God is first in our lives. God told Abraham to sacrifice his son on an altar, and although Isaac was Abraham's promised son, still he was obedient to God and God blessed him: "'Do not lay a hand on the boy,' he said. "Do not do anything to him. Now I know that you fear God, because you have not withheld from me your son, your only son'" (Genesis 22:12 NIV). That was Abraham's heart: he loved and revered the Lord more than his own son.

5

PEACE OF MIND

You will keep him in perfect peace,
Whose mind is stayed on You,
Because he trusts in You.

—Isaiah 26:3 (NKJV)

And they come to Jesus, and see him that was possessed
with the devil, and had the legion, sitting, and clothed,
and in his right mind: and they were afraid.

—Mark 5:15

How does one define peace of mind and heart? With so much trouble in this world, we are concerned and troubled by many things that are happening in our world. Conflicts between political parties, widespread natural disasters, wars and conflicts between countries, and the moral decline of our country can disturb many, and rightfully so. We live in a society where we are concerned about our children's welfare in education, the environment in which we raise them, and their future. How will we be able to invest in their future? People are worried!

Think for a moment, we can listen to the media and get caught up in the bad news we hear every day about what's going on around the world, and I can let those reports stir up all kinds of emotions: anger, fear, and anxiety. And for the rest of the day we are upset, can't sleep, and can't eat; we are troubled over things we can't control. Most of us think we can control what's going on in our society, and to a degree we can temporarily make changes for the better. When you see all of these things happening, what do you do? What is your mind-set? What is your perspective on how you view peace when there is so much chaos and trouble in this world? You will get a wide variety of opinions. Most people feel that they have the answers, but in most cases, those answers will come from some secular, educated, or political point of view.

Mind-set means the thought processes that you have allowed to govern the way you conduct yourself in life. It also has a bearing on your perspective on the issues and concerns we are all faced with every day. When you go to work, you are in a work mode to do your job to the best of your ability. When you go to a gym, you are in an exercise mode to improve your health. When you are at home cooking, you are in a mood to prepare meals and to make sure that the food is seasoned right, that the ingredients are right for certain dishes, and that the food is cooked on time. All these tasks require a conscious effort on our part to do it the right way, bringing results, and your mind is focused on that task to completion. So you labor in these things, knowing that a paycheck will come at the end of the week, a healthier body over a period of time, or a delicious meal when it's ready. What's the goal? A positive result with benefits.

My point is that your mind-set dictates how you perform in life. When see so many people who mess up their lives with extramarital affairs, drugs, or some type of domestic crime, we say to ourselves, *What were they thinking?* Well, they weren't thinking. How many times have we seen young men with exceptional talent and the potential to be a great athlete end up in trouble with the law over some domestic violence or drugs? It's a dilemma because they are in trouble all the time, and it's the same old common issue. This sounds funny, but you see that it's a true statement when you understand the concept: "You can take the person out of the ghetto, but you can't take the ghetto out of the person." Their mind-set has made them that way because that's the environment in which they were raised. They have a ghetto mentality, and that's all they know. If someone doesn't educate them, they can't see a better way of living.

My pastor used an illustration in that we need to think big. He told us a story of his wife taking his nieces to the top of a hill so they could view the beautiful homes in the area, and they were fascinated at what they saw. She told them that they could have something like this, breaking the mind-set that you can achieve if you trust God and work hard. They were exposed to the right kind of things where they can learn a lesson about achievement. The thought that I had was that when we begin to educate our minds, we break the ignorant ghetto mentality.

People are suffering because they don't know or they haven't been exposed to the right kind of knowledge to advance themselves in life. My success came from the exposure to military life and technical schools that I've attended over twenty-eight years. The knowledge that I've gained was rewarding, and working for the Department of Defense was my dream. The point was that this didn't happen overnight; it took some work, training, and schooling to get where I am. I had a mind-set of wanting to achieve success in my career. The same way that you educate yourself in wanting to achieve success in life is the same way you should fill your mind with the knowledge of God for success in your spirit. It starts in the mind, but the mind and the heart must be renewed. The truth be told I have exposed my heart and mind to the wrong things and I saw where that got me in trouble!

Faith in the word of God brings peace of mind to the heart of the believer. When the knowledge of God is believed, there is a working knowledge of that word that becomes life to your spirit. You don't just quote declarations from the scriptures—you possess them. The life of those words becomes a part of your thinking, and faith in what you are thinking, activates a power that comes from faith in what God has said. That dynamic power is the same power that created everything; it's the same authoritative power that made the demons come out of a man. This same power from God's word is the only power that brings peace of mind. The word of God is extremely powerful!

To develop this type of mindset, you have to meditate on the word of God and have confidence in what it says. For example, consider this scripture in 2 Thessalonians 2:1–2: "Now we beseech you, brethren, by the coming of our Lord Jesus Christ, and by our gathering together unto him, That ye be not soon shaken in mind, or be troubled, neither by spirit, nor by word, nor by letter as from us, as that the day of Christ is at hand." Now, how do you let that verse get into your spirit? By meditating on that word until faith comes, and when faith comes, power is released to give you the confidence to stand and not be troubled. You have just developed your mind in believing what God has said, because the peace of God is a state of being. God's peace is absolutely indescribable to explain; it's just believed and experienced through the work of faith.

When people around us are worried sick about the economy, conflict in the world, and many other problems and issues that affect our society, it is up to us as Bible believers to stand on the truth of God's word. Why? Because we know what's keeping us, and it's the promises of the word of God. Isaiah 26:2–3 says: "Open ye the gates, that the righteous nation which keepeth the truth may enter in. Thou wilt keep him in perfect peace, whose mind is stayed on thee: because he trusteth in thee." What a promise! You keep your mind on Jesus, and he will keep your mind at peace.

But it comes with conditions; clearly it doesn't fall on just anybody, because some people don't have peace. Notice the words *keepth* and *trusteth*; if you see these words with the "th" on the end, it means you continue to keep the truth and trust in God for the rest of your life. You don't fall away from the faith; you don't give up on what God promised you. You keep his word with all your might; he will keep you with all his might. Some people are trusting in things, and God blesses us with things to enjoy, but we can easily miss the whole concept of the Christian life. It's not the issue, it's what you believe. Charles Stanley says: "The key element in true, lasting peace is the presence of God," which is supported by Isaiah 26:3.

We have a choice to be what we want to be, and great as God is, he will not trespass on your will. Jesus said it perfectly that it is your choice to come to him. In Matthew 11:28–29 (NIV) he says: "Come to me, all you who are weary and burdened, and I will give you rest. Take my yoke upon you and learn from me, for I am gentle and humble in heart, and you will find rest for your souls." The rest is cessation of work, exertion, or activity; it also means peace, ease, or refreshment resulting from sleep or the cessation of an activity. When a person is at rest, they are not worried or disturbed by anything because of their state of mind at that moment.

God wants to give us his peace that will take us into eternity, not the temporal peace that the world offers. God says not to worry about things; we just need to enter into his rest, but we have to know something about how to obtain that rest and peace of mind that God gives. A story in the gospel of Luke gives a very good description of what happens when one is focused on Jesus or else focused on things that don't matter.

> As Jesus and his disciples were on their way, he came to a village where a woman named Martha opened her home to him. She had a sister called Mary, who sat at the Lord's feet listening to what he said. But Martha was distracted by all the preparations that had to be made. She came to him and asked, "Lord, don't you care that my sister has left me to do the work by myself? Tell her to help me!"
>
> "Martha, Martha," the Lord answered, "You are worried and upset about many things, but few things are needed—or indeed only one. Mary has

chosen what is better, and it will not be taken away from her." (Luke 10:38–42 NIV)

Mary sat at the feet of Jesus, listening to what he had to say without a care in the world. She was focused on Jesus, and Martha was running around worried about everything else. Which one of them are you? When we are maturing in the Lord, we have sometimes reflected both Mary's and Martha's state of mind. Learning not to worry takes a consistent prayer life and study of the word of God. Notice that I mentioned both prayer and the word. When you pray, your prayer needs substance, and the only substance is the word of God.

How do I obtain the peace of God? Joshua 1:8 says to meditate on the word day and night. Meditating is a practice in which an individual trains the mind or induces a mode of consciousness, either one to realize some benefit. According to Wikipedia's definition; the term *meditation* refers to a broad variety of practices (much like the term *sports*) that includes techniques designed to promote relaxation, build internal energy or life force, and develop compassion-love, patience, generosity, and forgiveness. Let's make this applicable to our lives, starting right now. How do we do this? Is there a formula for obtaining the peace of God? The majority of churches today aren't teaching faith and how to make it applicable to our lives. On the other hand, some are sitting in churches, and they still don't believe it. So if faith is not being taught, how can they obtain faith? Making it even clearer, what are you hearing?

I will declare this statement to anybody: we can please God and obey God only by *faith*. There is something special about faith that God sees and moves on your behalf. The reason why I keep harping on this topic of faith is that the peace of God comes by faith. This is how it works; reading the Bible is totally different from hearing a word from the Lord. When you read the Bible and you meditate on it until you get a revelation or that scripture becomes life (*Rhema*), then it's a word from the Lord that enters your spirit. Then faith has come, because faith comes by hearing and hearing by the word of God. When you have faith, a power is released, and God activates his ability to perform whatever that word says on your behalf because it pleases him that you choose to trust him, and from that trust you have peace. "But without faith it is impossible to please Him, for he who comes to God must believe that He is, and that He is a rewarder of those who diligently seek Him" (Hebrews 11:6 NKJV).

> If any man teach otherwise, and consent not to wholesome words, even the words of our Lord Jesus Christ, and to the doctrine which is according to godliness; He is proud, knowing nothing, but doting about questions and strife of words, whereof cometh envy, strife, railings, evil surmising, Perverse disputing of men of corrupt minds, and destitute of the truth, supposing that gain is godliness: from such withdraw thyself. (1 Timothy 6:3–5)

If you decide to depart from the teachings of the Lord Jesus, this will be the outcome of your life because now you have no guidance and stability. The word of God will keep you from falling apart only when you believe it and obey it. I have seen people described in this passage of scripture who departed from the faith and ended up tormented by their own philosophy, and it's just deception and the work of the enemy, and they have no peace at all.

You determine the outcome of your life by how you think. Committing your thinking to be scriptural takes times and effort to develop your mind to a mind of peace. The power of God is the activation of the word by faith working in your life. So when it comes to peace, something has to happen to your mind and heart for peace to be effective in your spirit. When we look for God to bless us, we usually equate that with some monetary blessing. God wants to restore our minds and put them back in right standing with him. Remember what happened after Jesus delivered the man from demonic torment: he was clothed and in his right mind. There was a calm about him; he had the peace of mind that only Jesus could bring. The greatest blessing is that you can have peace with God through our Lord and Savior Jesus Christ. The blessing is peace at home, peace in your marriage, peace in your spirit.

Listen: you have to make the decision to have that in your life. God will not force his peace on you. One thing that I and my lovely wife have decided on is that we are not going to argue and tear each other down. We love each other, we support each other's goals, and we communicate with each other about our feelings. And we communicate the word of God to each other, and it builds us both up to love and support each other. That's why I have peace of mind, and when I go home, I go home to a home of peace. I love going home to my wife; she has brought a great calm to me, she compliments me, and we work at it to make it work. We also defend each other's integrity because we are one, and we understand that concept from principles that we have learned from the word of God.

Men, if you want the God kind of peace in your life, in your home, and in your marriage, ask God to teach you how to be a man of peace. The secret is it's your choice, and think about this for a moment: We set up thoughts in our mind to be stubborn, and we have successfully done that. What will happen if you put God's thoughts in your mind that come from his word? If you put bad thoughts in your mind, you become what you think. If you put God's word in your mind, you become what God says.

Look at this simple verse: "Great peace have they which love thy law: and nothing shall offend them" (Psalm 119:165). He didn't say merely *peace*; rather, he put emphasis on the kind of peace by saying *great peace*. But the peace is conditional: you love his law—in other words, you love the word of God—and God grants you his peace because you love and obey his word. Becoming spiritually minded takes a commitment to thinking about what God says.

People can say all kinds of things about you, but what is your mind-set? It's not what they say about you that matters. It's what you are thinking and how you react that matters. If you have the knowledge of God in you, you will react like God in a righteous way. The scripture you put in your spirit will make the difference and the outcome of how things will work in your life. People are going to offend you, lie about you, and try to create trouble in your life. This can disturb your peace if you let it.

So how do you think? What's in your mind that will bring peace in your mind? Now, God said in his word that if you meditate on his word you will have good success and be prosperous (Joshua 1:8). Here comes the application part: find scriptures that deal with the promise of peace, and put your faith and confidence in those scriptures. Faith that is activated will energize your spirit to perform just like Jesus. Jesus said, "Without me, you can do nothing" (see John 15:5), so it's his power that is putting your mind at peace in the midst of the trouble. People will be amazed that nothing affects you, and they'll look at you and wonder how on earth you are laughing and smiling with no care in the world about the situation you are in. You have operated with a mindset based on the word of God; that's giving you this peace.

Here are the scriptures of promise that God gives us: "Be still, and know that I am God; I will be exalted among the nations, I will be exalted in the earth" (Psalm 46:10 NIV). "The Lord will fight for you, and you shall hold your peace and remain at rest" (Exodus 14:14 AMP). "Dearly beloved, avenge not yourselves, but rather give place unto wrath: for it is written, Vengeance is mine; I will repay, saith the Lord" (Romans 12:19).

You move in what you believe, based on what you've heard, and God will support you 100 percent. You can count on it! Faith in that will bring peace in your mind. You will not be troubled or disturbed because you have the knowledge of God working inside you, and it is dwelling in you richly. As the scripture says: "Let the word of Christ dwell in you richly in all wisdom; teaching and admonishing one another in psalms and hymns and spiritual songs, singing with grace in your hearts to the Lord" (Colossians 3:16). This is how you deal with life's battles and issues that face us each day. God has given us promises to stand on, and no person on this earth can defeat you.

To have his peace, you must know something. Paul told us to think about whatever is true, noble, just, pure, and lovely. What's true? Jesus is truth. What's noble? Jesus is noble! What's just? Jesus is just! What's pure? Jesus is pure! What's lovely? Jesus is lovely! All we need is faith in the Prince of Peace. Develop your mind in this way of thinking, and I guarantee that if you work this concept of believing in your spirit, you will experience a peace that you can't describe. As the scripture says, it passes all understanding, and you can't describe it because God made it so priceless and awesome. All you want to do is praise and worship him because he is the source of our peace. What an awesome King we serve!

6

EXERCISING YOUR FAITH

But strong meat belongs to them that are of full age,
even those who by reason of use have their senses
exercised to discern both good and evil.

—Hebrews 5:14

But you, dear friends, [build] yourselves up in your
most holy faith and [pray] in the Holy Spirit.

—Jude 1:20 (NIV)

My wife and I had a good conversation about the subject of faith
in God. Then a question came to my mind about the dynamics of
having faith. I asked her, "What is it about faith that pleases God
so much?"

The answer was very simple. After she thought about it for a
moment, she answered, "It's your choice to believe him because
he gives us the chance to choose." When we make that choice to
follow him, we have peace in what he promised us. It's like when
God appeared to Abraham and gave him a promise that he would
multiply his seed and bless his offspring; Abraham made a choice
to believe when he didn't see any evidence of what he believed. He
only heard a promised word from the Lord. He chose to believe that

God was who he said he was, and that moved God to the point that he made Abraham a righteous man. To take it a step further, the scriptures said that he became the friend of God (James 2:23). What a blessing that your faith can deepen your relationship with God to the point that God calls you his friend.

Not only was this done by faith alone, but also by obedience to the voice of the Lord. There was action to Abraham's faith in God. God told Abraham, "Go and leave this country and I'm going to bless you and your family and make you a prosperous man" (see Genesis 12:1). Abraham exercised his faith in God's spoken promise. The scripture teaches that we need to have the same faithful attitude as Abraham, who was called the father of faith.

When we say that we need to exercise our faith, what are we talking about? Exercise is the physical exertion of the body—making the body do a physical activity which results in a healthier level of fitness and both physical and mental over a period of time. Exercise is any continuous repetition of an activity to achieve some level of success. To achieve this level of fitness takes time, discipline, and commitment to a fitness program or some type of training, whether it's physical or mental, to achieve such results. Most people begin to see the benefits of exercise, and they come to enjoy its benefits to the point that it becomes a way of life for them. This type of activity promotes health in other areas of their lives as well.

What is faith in the simplest terms? Faith is complete trust or confidence in someone or something. It is a strong belief in God or in the doctrines of a religion, based on spiritual apprehension rather than proof. When you exercise, you develop strength and conditioning; in other words, you must put in some work to build up to that level of fitness. It's the same way spiritually: when you exercise your faith in the word of God, you are developing your faith in him. God has given us a measure of faith, and it is up to us to develop our faith. To put it another way, God has made all of us with muscles, and if you want to have an athletic build or be a bodybuilder, you have to develop your muscles through consistent training to get the results you desire. God is the same way about his word, in that we all have a measure of faith for us to develop. That's why some believers don't excel as others do, because they don't have a working knowledge of faith in their lives, and they haven't been taught how to develop their faith. I remember failing because I lacked the discipline to develop a working knowledge myself and it's not a good feeling. I felt like a failure because of my disobedience to God's Word.

To be an effective athlete, you have to train effectively by developing a good work ethic to maximize your performance. One thing athletes do is see what they need to work on in the off-season. Michael Jordan was perhaps the greatest basketball player, and I was always inspired by his work ethic to get better. He was talented and gifted to play the sport, but he lacked the strength to be competitive. He evaluated himself physically, and he began to incorporate a weight training program to perform at his best. It was so effective that he simply dominated the league. He won six NBA championships and several scoring titles, becoming one of the greatest players in NBA history. He applied himself to get better and develop the skill to be better.

How are we to examine ourselves to see where we are? We have to start where we are to see what we need to do to develop ourselves in the word of God, just as Jordan evaluated his strengths and weaknesses and then worked on strengthening his weaknesses and continued to polish his strengths, making himself a formidable opponent to guard. God sees you no differently than he does the next person. You have a measure of faith given to you; then it's up to you to develop it. You have to take advantage of the opportunities given to you to develop yourself and exercise your faith in the things of God. This scripture makes clear the desire of the believer: "But without faith it is impossible to please Him, for he who comes to God must believe that He is, and that He is a rewarder of those who diligently seek Him" (Hebrews 11:6 NKJV). It takes patience to be developed, and God is a God of patience in developing you in him. We don't try to force our children to grow up fast; they must be nurtured as they grow.

The other thing about growth is that it may hurt a little while you are growing in faith. Jesus said, "Upon this rock I will build my church" (Matthew 16:18). How does he build his church? Christ's words of faith are the building blocks for developing your faith. Developing your faith takes consistent effort, and like the scripture says, you diligently seek him every day. You can't work out one day and say that you are in good shape; it doesn't work that way. Faith alone will not work; it takes faith and obedience. In other words, you must move in what you believe. Abraham heard and responded: he believed what he heard, and he moved. The God told him to leave his country and promised to show him a land of blessing.

In today's world we are bombarded with so much that it has become difficult for the average believer to really respond in faith. The exposure of healthy biblical teaching is the key to building a body of believers in the word of God where their faith can be developed. How do people stay the same when they hear the teaching of the word week after week? How do they leave the presence of an anointed word of God and don't change their behavior? What in the world are they hearing? If it sounds as if I'm describing the profile of how most church people are, you are right. I am very concerned with the welfare and the health of believers. We should all have a passion to move by faith; it is the hallmark of our walk with God.

What you need to do is have a hunger and a desire for the word of God so that you can hear a word of faith to bless your spirit. Become spiritually proactive in your quest for teaching, studying, and applying the principles found in the word of God. Your faith is exercised by what you know and what you've practiced. You begin to build yourself up in faith, and you reach a level of maturity in the faith. Yes, it's a faith walk, but it is also an application of that faith that makes the difference. God wants the best for us, and yes, there will be trials and troubles that will affect us all, but we have faith in God to help us through them.

When you exercise your faith daily, it's just like putting your body through an exercise program. All the exercises cause exertion of the muscles over a period of time, and the muscles become conditioned. During the process of exercising your faith, you become what I call "faith conditioned." Athletes in the off-season go through a weight training program and a conditioning program, getting the body ready to be competitive in their sport because of the constant pounding the body will go through in a game or competition.

Sometimes teams will physically dominate a team with their strength, speed, power, and intelligence. If the other team is not ready for it, they will be defeated because they lack the abilities to make themselves successful. The same thing applies to us spiritually; if we don't exercise our spiritual muscles in the word of God, we can take a beating from the enemy or from life's problems and issues because we lack the spiritual strength to stand. How do you build spiritual strength? You learn from the people who are strong spiritually in faith. I remember failing because I lacked the discipline to develop a working knowledge myself and it's not a good feeling. I felt like a failure because of my disobedience to God's Word.

How does one build muscle? Someone who is a bodybuilder will show you the right techniques to build strength the right way. The more you associate yourself with weight lifters daily; you will begin to develop muscle like them. You will take on the characteristics of a bodybuilder's physique. They will also show you how to eat the right foods for optimal results. So you have to be taught and trained so it can be affective for you to develop the right way. The wrong concepts of faith have been taught in churches, and people start out in error spiritually. This can be done the right way, and it will take the process to change your mind from erroneous concepts and ways of thinking. When you believe the right way, you will get the right results. When you believe the wrong way, you will get the wrong result.

Building strength in God takes time, and he is rich in patience in developing you in his word. I remember when I started to incorporate squats in my exercise program, and I quickly realized how weak my legs were. So week after week I would perform these different squat exercises, working every angle of the leg for overall muscle development and strength. I was extremely sore afterward, taking up to three days to recover. One day I realized that the weight was becoming easier to lift, and I didn't get quite as sore. I gave myself a strength test to see if I'd made some improvement. When I started, I could only squat 75 pounds—sad but true. Later, I tested myself one day, and I squatted 225 pounds easily. I could tell the difference in my running and overall strength. Sometimes building is hard labor, and it hurts, but it's necessary for growth, and we become equipped through the exercising of faith to strengthen others in what we have learned.

Jesus told Peter (Luke 22:31) that Satan desired to destroy him—as Jesus put it, "that he may sift you like wheat." But Jesus encouraged him and said, "But I have prayed for you, Simon, that your faith may not fail. And when you have turned back, strengthen your brothers" (Luke 22:32 NIV). In the King James Version he said, "When thou art converted, strengthen thy brethren." So that lets us know that God will give us his power to stand when we are converted.

Power comes from Jesus through the work of the Holy Spirit which causes us to enhance our faith and walk with the Lord. The spiritual rebirth increases our capacity to receive the word of faith from God's word. There has to be a reconstruction of our thinking because we first have to tear down bad thinking patterns that have plagued the human mind for years. We are by nature creatures of habit; that habit is rooted deep within us, and it's hard for us to change the way we do things. When we live a life of believing and exercising our faith in the word of God, something is happening to us on the inside. There is a change in our mind and spirit because we have allowed God to invade our thinking with his word.

Are you developing yourself in the word of God? I can't make the call on your life; you should know. Have you ever evaluated yourself? Are you walking in faith? Paul puts it this way: "Examine yourselves to see whether you are in the faith; test yourselves. Do you not realize that Christ Jesus is in you—unless, of course, you fail the test?" (2 Corinthians 13:5 NIV). Many Christians find themselves in their predicament because, as F. F. Bosworth said, "Most Christians feed their bodies three hot meals a day and their spirit one cold snack a week. And they wonder why they're so weak in faith." That's why we don't get the victory over life's battles; we're not exercising faith to strengthen ourselves.

You have to start where you are if you want to grow. Nobody can build a house starting with the roof; you start at the foundation. The foundation has to harden and be stable to build upon. Watching concrete dry and harden is boring, but it's necessary for growth to be effective, If the foundation is not solid, what will the structure look like?

Jesus is the author and finisher of our faith, and he is the foundation of our faith. He is the master builder of our faith, and all we have to do is cooperate with his program of exercising our faith, and he builds us up in him. We become pillars of faith for his purpose, and he qualifies us to work for him. We are no different from the apostles; they were just like us, but God poured his grace on them to preach the kingdom. They were so effective that the scriptures said that they turned the world upside down, according to Acts 17:6. We can be just like them, being rooted and build up in the word of God, because we have exercised our faith in the word of God.

7

ENJOYING YOUR LIFE

Command those who are rich in this present world not
to be arrogant nor to put their hope in wealth, which is
so uncertain, but to put their hope in God, who richly
provides us with everything for our enjoyment.

—1 Timothy 6:17 (NIV)

Enjoying your life is a privilege that most people don't have,
either because they were brought up in a certain lifestyle or because
they are ignorant of the better lifestyle and can't obtain it. We choose
the way we want to live, and either we deal with the consequences of
our poor choices, or we benefit from the decision we make in life to
improve ourselves. Many times we come across people who've never
been on a vacation, who've never gone out to eat at a nice restaurant,
or who've never exposed themselves to just the simple things in life.
To make this practical, the way we view life is determined by our
perspective on how we want to live, whether it's good or not. You
have the choice to make your life enjoyable.

Having a wonderful life is the result of your doing something
positive that's causing you to be that way. In order for us to reach the
goal of having this type of lifestyle, we have to make little changes
in the ways we do things every day. The classical saying that we all

have heard is "Insanity: is doing the same thing over and over again and expecting different results." That's one of our problems in how we manage our lives. To break that cycle, we need to break our way of thinking.

To be on your way to a happy, peaceful, enjoyable life, where does it start? It starts with you! The changes that you make in your mind is where it starts. Everybody that has made major changes in their life for the better has first made a change of mind and a change of heart. They've practiced little healthy habits and ethics to see them improve their life. The most powerful thing you have is your mind and the freedom to choose how you want to live. I used to be concerned with people that live on the streets and under bridges and I wonder how they ended up in a situation like that. I know that they made bad decisions and didn't exercise wisdom in certain areas, but who hasn't? I know I've made some awful decisions; we all have, with consequences that cost us a lot. But to see them totally give up on life and live in the streets makes me realize most of them chose to live that kind of lifestyle. Are we any better than them? No, it's a choice!

When we take a view of life, we need to look at certain elements that make up our lifestyle. In this last chapter I want you to try to change your way of thinking of just sitting down for a few minutes, looking at your life, and finding out why you are not happy. Here are some questions to think about when you really take a good look at yourself. You need to look at each question and answer them honestly to yourself. I will give you a hint. "My people are destroyed for the lack of knowledge" should be a good start. I promise you that every question below has a scriptural answer to that problem, and it's not just the scripture; it's faith in what it says that causes it to be a working knowledge in your life. To put it in other words, you need to develop a working knowledge of that scripture in your spirit. Think about these questions:

Why don't I have fulfillment in my life?
What am I doing with my life?

How did I get myself in this mess? (A classic one!)
(For any unhappy singles) Why I'm not married?
Why am I having financial problems?
Why am I having problems in my marriage?
Why can't I achieve a goal?
Why do I associate with people who can't benefit
me spiritually and physically?
Where are my morals and values? Where do I draw
the line?
What life is better than the life God has to offer?
Please! Somebody tell me!
Why am I so mean? Why am I hard to love?
Nobody wants to be around me—why?

For us to get to where we're living a joyous life, we need to be confronted with the truth of the word of God. Jesus said, "You shall know the truth and the truth will make you free" (John 8:32 NKJV). The best way to start is to recognize where you are, and it starts with a self-examination. You'll be surprised when you sit down and simply think.... Now just put down this book for a moment and think about the life God wants you to have. Ask yourself the tough questions. Some of you should be in tears, and let me be personal and up front with you—I certainly was!

"Lord, my life is a mess, and I can't enjoy anything. What is my problem?" The only thing that was coming out of me was frustration, and as T. D. Jakes once said, it was the silent screams that nobody heard, or at least that's what I thought. Why? Because I was overwhelmed with failure and guilt, and I was out of step with God's principles. It wasn't that God's principles weren't with me; it was because I ignored them, thinking that I knew something better than what God has to offer, and the result of my thinking made me a disobedient child.

So I went through a kind of prodigal son experience. I could talk about all the problems that I went through, but I want to wrap it up with this statement: it was a sin and out of the will of God, and

I wasn't happy. The scripture says the way of a transgressor is hard (Proverbs 13:15). When you live a life of disobedience, you will suffer the consequences of your actions, and sometimes they can become severe and tragic because you are out of the will of God. God has a way of getting our attention when we are out of line, and sometimes we need to be reminded that God is a God of love, but he is also our heavenly Father who corrects us when we need it. It may seem severe when the correction comes, but it's under grace and his love for us. God has given us his word because he wants us to have the best. He wants us to succeed in life and have victory over the enemy and other circumstances that come against us every day. Read this passage of scripture about how concerned, God is for us to be like his Son:

> "... Because the Lord disciplines the one he loves,
> and he chastens everyone he accepts as his son."

> Endure hardship as discipline; God is treating you as his children. For what children are not disciplined by their father? If you are not disciplined—and everyone undergoes discipline—then you are not legitimate, not true sons and daughters at all. Moreover, we have all had human fathers who disciplined us and we respected them for it. How much more should we submit to the Father of spirits and live! They disciplined us for a little while as they thought best; but God disciplines us for our good, in order that we may share in his holiness. No discipline seems pleasant at the time, but painful. Later on, however, it produces a harvest of righteousness and peace for those who have been trained by it. (Hebrews 12:6–11 NIV)

This sounds tough, but sometimes the tough discipline of the Lord is necessary for us to grow up to be mature. For us to face the truth, we have to acknowledge where we are; only when you find this out will you realize how far off you are. I know this sounds rough, but my life is a life of happiness because I went through the tough grind of exercising my faith in the word of God. I'm trying to help you be delivered from yourself and get you to see, as the old show said, that "Father Knows Best." I didn't like it, but I didn't complain. I just knew I was in a mess, and I sought the counsel of the Lord for help. After you have done some soul-searching, finding that you need the Lord to help you, then the healing can begin. The deliverance is on the way. It all comes through the application of knowledge that is worked by faith in the Lord's power to strengthen you.

Our task as believers is to study and search diligently until we have discovered the principle of what God is telling us. For example, the unjust steward in Luke 16 made bad decisions and wasted his master's goods. But the steward saw his error and did something about it. The scriptures said he went to all of his master's debtors and negotiated their debts down to a manageable level. What I like about this passage of scripture is that Jesus said that the master commended him for how he had dealt with the debtors.

The principle in this scripture reminds me of the time I had to owe money to my creditors. Being very irresponsible caused me a lot of problems, and I couldn't enjoy my life because of my poor management of finances. The worst feeling was that my paycheck wasn't mine; it belonged to somebody else. Frustrated and upset with myself, I had to sit down and listen to God. I said, "Lord, I can't live like this. I will never be able to enjoy my life if I continue this cycle of being irresponsible."

I had the "rob Peter to pay Paul" mentality, and it was absolutely horrible. A lot of factors had an impact on my problem; they included ignorance of how to manage my finances, disobedience to the word of God, and not making enough money. I was just simply limited in resources to recover from my situation. I simply said, "Lord, help me," and by his grace and mercy he did and much more.

Finally, I landed a very good job working for the government. I asked for wisdom and understanding in financial matters, and the Lord led me to read and hear seminars from well-known people like Dave Ramsey, Suze Orman, and the late Larry Burkett that have impacted and changed my way of thinking about money. The Bible says, among a multitude of counselors there is safety (see Proverbs 15:22). If you want to be financially blessed and successful, these are the sort of counselors you need to be listening to— or better yet, find the books they have written and make them a part of your library to enhance your understanding about financial matters.

The lesson I learned is that when you find out you are doing things that are not right, talk to people who are successful in the area that you're dealing with. This is just an example; the lesson applies to dealing with any issue in your life, whether in your marriage, home, finances, or health. There are experts in these matters that you can seek out. They became successful through trials and mistakes too, but they learned from them. Success is not just getting it right all the time; it's also learning from mistakes. Those who have done so can tell you the pitfalls to avoid because of their experience.

When seeking a better way to live, find the people who are living that type of lifestyle, and learn from them. You want a good marriage; find a couple that has a good relationship. You want to be financially successful; find a person who's done well in financial matters such as a broker or an investor. To work on bodily health, find a person in good physical shape and very healthy.

Find individuals that are spiritually minded in the things of God. Find people who operate in faith. When you apply the principles they teach you, your life will be enhanced, and you will start to live better. When we tithe and give liberal offerings to the church we support, God blesses our finances and gives us wisdom to manage what we make, and my wife and I enjoy the blessings of following God's principles of sowing and reaping.

Before I was married, the Lord established me in his principles, and I live a life of harmony in the Lord. Then after about a year the Lord's timing led me to meet my wife, who had it together when we met. The hand of God was on our marriage and still is, because we both knew that this was the right time and it was right in our spirit. Yes, I was financially, spiritually, and morally damaged due to my own spiritual negligence and ignorance. But the grace and mercy of God that I experienced can't be explained in words; all I can do is praise and worship him because he is too good. I just clamped down and obeyed his principles. This testimony may speak to you, and it may or may not be that severe, but I know for sure that there is something in your life you want to see fulfilled. What is it?

I remember one day the word of the Lord came to me when he was dealing with me about a promise to me. He said, "If you walk upright before me, I will not withhold any good thing from you." The best thing that he promised me was manifested when I found my wife. The scriptures say, "He who finds a wife finds what is good and receives favor from the LORD" (Proverbs 18:22 NIV). There is nothing more fulfilling than serving the Lord Jesus, marrying the queen of my heart, and being a daddy to my lovely daughters. In that order those are my priorities in life. If you want to enjoy your life, make it your priority to put God first in your life. There are people right in our congregations who put on a front, and their home life and marriage is horrible. You can obviously see the anguish on their faces, and it tells the whole story about what's going on at home. Exposure to the teachings is one thing, but the application of that teaching is another. How you apply the word to your life has an impact on how it affects your life.

Following the principles of God in the scriptures is the hallmark of having an enjoyable life. But the added benefit of this working successfully in your life is the work of the Holy Ghost in your life. Your life needs changes if you want to enjoy a new way of living. The apostles' lives were impacted by the teachings of Jesus as well as their spiritual conversion when they experienced the baptism of the Holy Spirit which transformed their lives. Jesus promised this to them, and after they received the Holy Spirit, their lives were different, and they enjoyed the new life they were living. The scriptures explain in detail the events after the day of Pentecost, and I want you to see that it was attractive enough to be noticed by the people, so that some received the preaching of Jesus and they believed and were changed by the power of the Holy Spirit. Something happened to the apostles, who changed from a scared and intimidated group of men to powerful men of God who spoke and proclaimed the resurrection of Jesus. Let's read the scripture text below to get an insight on what happened after Pentecost:

> Then they that gladly received his word were baptized: and the same day there were added unto them about three thousand souls. And they continued steadfastly in the apostles' doctrine and fellowship, and in breaking of bread, and in prayers. And fear came upon every soul: and many wonders and signs were done by the apostles. And all that believed were together, and had all things common; and sold their possessions and goods, and parted them to all men, as every man had need. And they, continuing daily with one accord in the temple, and breaking bread from house to house, did eat their meat with gladness and singleness of heart, praising God, and having favor with all the people. And the Lord added to the church daily such as should be saved. (Acts 2:41–47)

This passage of scripture gives much evidence that they enjoyed this new life that they were experiencing. Some of the people were afraid of them and in awe at how the Lord had transformed them. That's the beauty of the gospel: when it's believed, it has the power to change your life. To enjoy this type of living, you need to practice exercising your faith in the principles that come from the word of God. I have recently done a study about building yourself spiritually, and I concluded that you make yourself every day, whether you are conscious of it or not. Just by the pattern of thinking and the habits you practice, there is an end result of your actions and behavior. When you start making those little changes in your thinking, you make little changes in how you do things. This is how your life is changed for the better.

When you learn a concept from the word of God and you comprehend that concept, now you have information that is useful and applicable to your life. When I studied the concept about the unjust steward, I saw me and I saw how irresponsible I was and my thinking needed to be changed because it was affecting my life. Having no wisdom in financial matters makes life difficult and it affects your lifestyle because you can't do anything. Every creditor is after your money and you can't enjoy life like that until you change how you view money. My change came through the teaching on how to get back on financial track. The word of God says it this way: "Wisdom is the principal thing; therefore get wisdom: and with all thy getting get understanding" (Proverbs 4:7 KJV). I'm using finances as an example to whatever issue that you are coming up short on. There is something in all of our lives that we can do better if we would seek God in prayer to give us the knowledge and wisdom in his word to apply to whatever problem we have and we will be successful in life. The impact of this has great rewards, you become something in God. A man by the name of Frank Outlaw Late President of the Bi-Lo Stores made this famous quote that is very insightful:

> "Watch your thoughts, they become words;
> watch your words, they become actions;
> watch your actions, they become habits;
> watch your habits, they become character;
> watch your character, for it becomes your destiny."

Changes start with a thought and thoughts need to be the word of God. Your thinking can bring great rewards or they can get you in a world of trouble which ultimately leads to your destiny. Look at the first quote thoughts and words, what if your thoughts are

God's thoughts and what if your words are God's words. What will be the outcome of your actions, habits, character and destiny? If it's the word of God is involved in the equation the outcome will be a wonderful, peaceful, righteous life. You have to build your character based on practicing the fundamental truths of the word of God. Making this concept apart of your life will lead to a godly lifestyle and success. If God wants us to be holy like he is holy, then he wants us to live like him. Sometimes we need to start at ground zero and see the errors we made in our lives and completely start all over.

We need a total makeover in all areas of our lives. I'm telling you I did, and I want you to remember that once you start developing yourself in the discipline of applying the word, it's not easy. It's difficult at times because it's putting you in an uncomfortable situation that you are not used to. A change makes all of us uncomfortable, but it's necessary. Think about what's being done to you, and it's for the better. Introducing your body to a hard workout that you've never done before in the gym will make you sore if it's done effectively, but it yields great benefits to your physical condition. Sometimes you are so sore because your body is not used to it. It's the same way with life; sometimes we need to go through tough training and learn some tough lessons, whether they are spiritual or physical, for us to learn how to live a life that's pleasing to God. Most people today live better because of the lessons they've learned from their mistakes. There's nothing more wonderful than waking up with the peace of God in your life. We are faced with the challenges and trials of life, but the Lord teaches us how to have a godly mind-set about any situation that arises in our lives.

We have to have faith in what God has promised in his word. I want to make this crucial statement relevant to our lives as Christians: we must not only have faith, we must have a working knowledge of that faith. In other words, we must apply it. If there is no application of the knowledge of the word, there will be no success in life. The opposite of success is failure, and when you don't have the knowledge, you lack the ability to move forward in life.

We need information as much as we need inspiration. Remember, I mentioned balance. Inspiration is needful and has its place, but information is priceless, and it's applicable to everyday living. People who enjoy their life are thinking with an open mind, and they view life with a humble spirit.

Here are some statements to think about. They can put you in the right mind-set to think about yourself and how you view life. I call them "thoughts to live by":

- ❖ God is on your side. He's your Lord, he loves you, and he will reward you.
- ❖ God is your source for happiness, peace, and joy.
- ❖ Be thankful to the Lord for all that he has done for you.
- ❖ Be obedient to the Lord.
- ❖ Ask God to help you with life's issues.
- ❖ Develop and work on your marriage, and be romantic in the little things. Love on each other with all your heart.
- ❖ Learn to stop being unpleasant and evil to people for no reason. God sees it!
- ❖ Learn to love people.
- ❖ Learn to keep quiet sometimes.
- ❖ Learn to celebrate people.
- ❖ Stop complaining about the little things that don't matter.
- ❖ Have a heart to learn.
- ❖ Be adventurous, travel, and see the world. God made the world, not just your little city.
- ❖ Stop taking advantage of people's goodness.
- ❖ It's okay not to know everything. That's why learning is stimulating and interesting; it shows that there are some things you don't know, and that's okay.
- ❖ Have fun, and be a kid at heart sometimes.
- ❖ Laugh, and laugh loud! There's nothing like a good, gut-wrenching, laugh that brings tears to your eyes. It's good for you, and it's contagious.

❖ Quit thinking you are too cute and mature to have fun.

❖ Get some balance in your life.

❖ Don't take yourself too seriously, but take God very seriously.

❖ Stop being a racist—that's all of us—because you never know who you will need.

❖ Keep things simple. Don't complicate things.

❖ Work on your attitude. Attitude determines altitude.

❖ Leave people alone. Don't be bothersome to people.

❖ Don't wait until tragedy strikes for you realize the importance of life and family.

❖ Don't be afraid to take some risk, depending on what it is.

❖ Not everybody is like you.

❖ Keep an open mind.

❖ Rest your body and mind. Have a lazy day!

❖ Have a junk food day! (I love those days!)

❖ When trusting God, expect him to see you through.

❖ When all this is over and you come to end of your life, always remember that Jesus loves you, and he is coming again!

These types of thoughts have allowed me to keep everything in perspective when it comes to living a life that's enjoyable. It may not be joyful all the time because of the situations we are faced with from time to time. But when we develop a working knowledge of the word of God in our lives, then our life is affected by his power to overcome whatever comes against us. Think about the things of God, and move in them, and watch them impact your life. Jesus made an encouraging statement regarding us he said: "Fear not, little flock; for it is your Father's good pleasure to give you the kingdom" (Luke 12:32). The kingdom is in us, which means the ruling of God's principles dwells within you to bless you and make you a blessing to others.

We don't need to be afraid of life; we need to have victory over our life. God wants us to live an abundant life that comes from him, and we need to make it attractive for people to come to him. We are the body of Christ that represents and expresses who he is. Don't just preach and bring the lost to church; let them see your life, and let it be winsome. Win them over by how you live, not what you say.

When Jesus walked this earth, his life attracted people; some loved him, and others hated him. But it could not be ignored either by the religious sects or the common people of that day. The scripture text says that "immediately His fame spread throughout all the region around Galilee" (Mark 1:28 NKJV). Why was he well-known to the community? He went to people that needed him. He loved people, and people loved him. He was a very humble man, not proud and arrogant, and they were attracted to him. In other words, he was very approachable and made people feel comfortable around him. If anybody can pick up on a person's nature and attitude, definitely children can. They were always attracted to him, and I believe they were like kids today: they love to get in your face, and they were intrigued by this man. He had an attractive charisma about him that the religious sects envied. His life is an example to show us how to walk like he walked.

Jesus lived a life that was absolutely impeccable, and the religious leaders of that day took notice of it, and it intimidated them. What does that say about us? Well, your life can have an impact on people, whether they like you or not. It doesn't matter; it's the principle of the way we live and conduct our lives in the presence of people with whom we associate daily. We need to get away from putting on a pompous religious act of living and keep it biblical in application and simple in the fundamental principles on how to live. Jesus' life was not complicated; it was simple in nature and spiritual in reality and application. No matter what is going on in your life, I want to encourage you that you can improve your life. The resources are out there for you to be able to achieve results. When I had the issues with my finances, I went to the seminars and received some good information how to manage what I make.

God has put people in our lives who have excelled in areas that we need to excel in. For students to excel in school, they need to listen and learn from an instructor that is knowledgeable in that area where they want to be successful. It's the same way with life when it comes to the desire to live right and manage your life the way God intended. Some of you will start out feeling this hurts, and it feels uncomfortable to change the way you do things, but we are built with the ability to adapt under pressure. This is where God can do his work in us when we are at ground zero, and being built hurts sometimes, but stay with it because it is so rewarding when you submit to the disciplines of God's blessings.

I want to show you what God will do if you let him into your heart to get your life in order. He promises you something in his word after you have been through some of the difficult trials of life: "But the God of all grace, who hath called us unto his eternal glory by Christ Jesus, after that ye have suffered a while, make you perfect, stablish, strengthen, settle you" (1 Peter 5:10). God is making us into the image of his Son by transforming our spirit and will establish his word in us when we submit to his instructions.

Our problem as believers is that we are not living the Spirit-filled life because we have not been taught correctly how to. The scripture says, "Grace and peace be multiplied unto you through the knowledge of God, and of Jesus our Lord, according as His divine power hath given unto us all things that pertain unto life and godliness, through the knowledge of Him that hath called us to glory and virtue" (2 Peter 1:2–3). Look at how the scripture starts out with grace and peace being multiplied in your life through the application of the knowledge of the word of God. He is calling us to a life of godliness that pleases him, and we have his divine authority (power) to live a wonderful life in Christ Jesus.

Your life can be wonderful when you trust in the living God. Jesus is the focus of our lives, and we are saved by his life. So we just need to believe it and walk in it. Is it that simple? No, it's not. I would be lying if I said it is. That's why God says in Hebrews that we must diligently seek him. Yes! It's a diligent walk. This walk is a walk of faith and prayer, focusing on the Lord Jesus who is our source of strength. We must develop a diligent mind and willing heart to walk with Jesus. This is the hallmark of every believer who wants to live a life of peace and joy in the Lord: they are growing closer to him. Keep striving to get to know him, and seek him. Don't just seek the kingdom, but seek the king of that kingdom. Jesus is the source of everything, and it comes from him and through him. Your faith in the word of God activates his gift of your ability to live an anointed life under the guidance and direction of the Holy Ghost.

We are to live a peaceful life, but also need to be spiritually vigilant against the world's philosophies. We must learn to keep everything in perspective, according to the knowledge of the word of God. The word of God is so dynamic that it can tailor to anybody's life and do a dynamic work on their spirit and impact their life. Sometimes these Christian claims can be dubious in the world, as if we are telling a fable, but it's not. It's just like loving your family: you can't explain it thoroughly, but you just know that you do, and you do things to show that love to them. Having the life of Christ in your spirit is the same way: you can't fully explain it, but many times you don't have to—you just have to live life with authenticity and let others see your life. They can't question the life if it's authentic.

That has been one of the churches' problems. We put on a show at church, but after we leave, we turn into something else other than showing the nature and the character of Christ. Jesus said, "Let your light so shine before men, that they may see your good works, and glorify your Father which is in heaven" (Matthew 5:16). He didn't say *your mouth*; he said *your light*, how your life is conducted before men. It's a life that people will be attracted to when they see the genuine peace and joy flowing from you. There will be an expression on your face that they can't explain, but they will know that it's something different, something special, and it's the life of Christ who is working through you. Your life is the greatest testimony you have, especially when they know what you used to be and see your life transformed into something wonderful. Eventually they will question why you conduct yourself as you do, and the opportunity will open a door to give them your testimony.

The scriptures include this passage to show us that we need to be set apart from how the world thinks and how they live: "But sanctify the Lord God in your hearts: and be ready always to give an answer to every man that asketh you a reason of the hope that is in you with meekness and fear" (1 Peter 3:15). Notice the word *sanctify*, which means to be set apart for God's purpose and to show the world we are different. Our lives will be examined by the world, and they will see the hope that is in us and wonder what it is about our character that's special.

True joy and peace come from having the Spirit of God simply working in your life to enhance your life. When you are delivered from the bondage of sin and have the peace of God residing in you, how can you not enjoy that? Jesus came to liberate the souls of humankind from the penalty and bondage of sin and put them in his body and his kingdom. He said it is his Father's pleasure to give us the kingdom, and what a kingdom we are going to get! But while we are still living in these bodies, we live a life of hope in the Lord because of what he promised us. Joy is based on faith in what God promised us, and no matter what happens in life—whether we face trials, tribulations, or even death, which seems to be so grim—we have an eternal hope in the Lord Jesus. Our joy is an eternal joy; our peace is an eternal peace because we look for our Savior to appear in all his splendor and glory from heaven. Even after we have lived a victorious life on this earth and we face death, we know that the best is yet to come because the Lord Jesus is coming for his church. Just imagine that the greatest man who ever lived (it's the greatest story ever told) and the only one raised from the dead with all power is coming for his people. Jesus is our joy, and he is our peace. Do you want to enjoy your life? Put your faith in the Lord Jesus, trust him with your life, give everything to him, and you will experience the true meaning of spiritual joy and peace that will nourish your soul and heart. Enjoy your life every day, and live each day with thanksgiving to the Lord.

Conclusion

In conclusion, I want to let every reader of this book know that I had one intention: to bless you with information that can be applied to your life. This book was inspired, and although I have completed this task, I had great joy and fun writing this book. I sincerely hope that you digested the spiritual meaning in each chapter and that this book can be a tool and a study help to impact your spiritual and natural life.

My greatest desire for you is that you live a life that has meaning and purpose. Developing our spiritual walk in personal study, prayer and devotion are a part of our lifestyle. Make sure that the information you read in this book should only be the beginning of your success, and strive to build on your success with more knowledge about being healthy spiritually and naturally. It's a mindset and an attitude that will determine that.

My lovely wife is the greatest example of God's love for me. We have declared the word of God over our marriage, our children, and our home, and the Lord has truly blessed our home to be peaceful and loving. That is a choice, and as with anything else, when it's done God's way, it's an attitude, according to God's way and success according to God's promises. Remember, you can go and preoccupy yourself with a lot of so-called church work, simply being too busy, and miss out on being successful at home. My wife and heard a statement that I want to share with you: "No amount of success can compensate for failure at home." You can do all of these other things, but if you are missing it at home, you haven't accomplished anything. Priorities don't begin at church, school, or any other institution; they start at home. A person's life is determined by their home life, not how they perform out in the world. Most people put on masks when they step out of their homes, and we have no idea how they live. How do you live? That's the challenge! Are we truly living for God in a way that brings honor to his name? These questions confronted and challenged me to do better and live better. That's my concern, and it inspired me to write this book for us to examine and take a good look at our lives to see if we are truly living this life God's way.

May the grace of God and our Savior, the Lord Jesus Christ, bless you in your quest to live the life that honors him and blesses others in their walk with the Lord. God has given us everything we need to live a life that's spiritually healthy and successful in him. Follow his kingdom principles, apply them to your life, and you will experience the peace and joy that he wants you to have. May God richly bless you!

References

Barker, Kenneth L., General editor (1995). *New International Version Study Bible.* Grand Rapids. MI: Zondervan Publishers

Bromiley, Geoffrey W., Editor (1979). *International Standard Bible Encyclopedia.* Grand Rapids, MI: William B. Eerdmans Publishing Co.

Kenneth Copeland Ministries, Inc. (1991). *King James Version Bible Reference Edition.* Ft. Worth, TX: Kenneth Copeland Ministries, Inc.

Merriam-Webster's Collegiate Dictionary, tenth edition

Strong, James, LL.D., S.T.D. (1990). *The New Strong's Exhaustive Concordance of the Bible.* Nashville, TN: Thomas Nelson Publishers Inc.

Unger, Merrill F. (1988). *Unger's Bible Dictionary.* Chicago. IL: Moody Press, c/o MLM.

Vine, W. E., William White Jr., And Merrill F. Unger, editors (1985). *Vine's Complete Expository Dictionary of Old and New Testament Words.* Nashville, TN: Thomas Nelson, Inc., Publishers.

Online Resources

Wikipedia (http://en.wikipedia.org/wiki/)
http://quoteinvestigator.com/2013/01/10/watch-your-thoughts
http://www.faithfull.org/teaching/source.htm

http://www.stempublishing.com/magazines/cf/1896/Wholesome-Words-Even-the-Words-Of-Our-Lord-Jesus-Christ.html "Wholesome Words, Even the Words of Our Lord Jesus Christ" http://thoroughlynourishedlife.com http://preceptaustin.org/ "Living Life More Abundantly", Charles E. Bryce. Enduring Church of God, Publishers of Straightforward Magazine

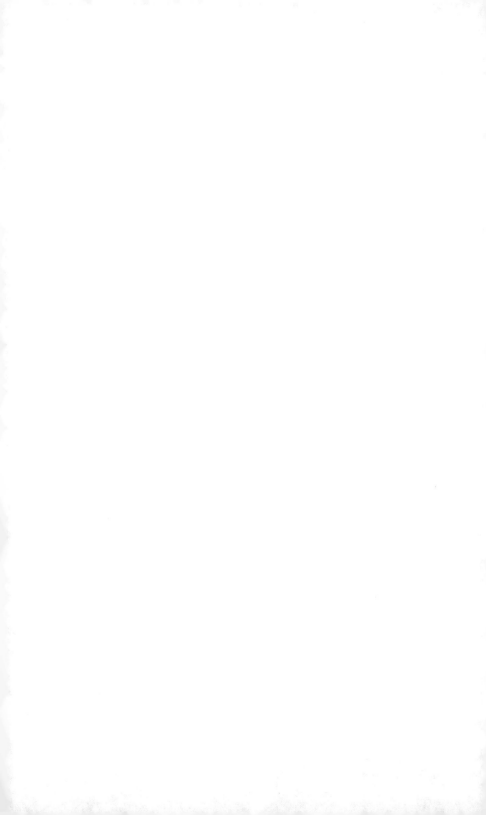

Printed in the United States
By Bookmasters